Yoga Journal's

YOGA BASICS

MARA CARRICO

and the Editors of *Yoga Journal*

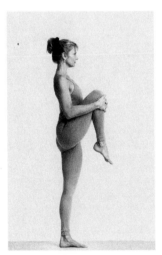 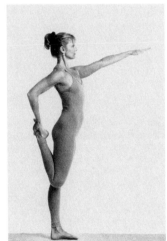 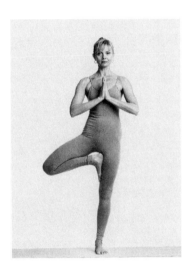

WITH 140 PHOTOGRAPHS

An Owl Book   Henry Holt and Company   New York

Yoga Journal's

YOGA

The Essential
Beginner's Guide to Yoga
for a Lifetime
of Health and Fitness

BASICS

Henry Holt and Company, Inc.
Publishers since 1866
115 West 18th Street
New York, New York 10011

Henry Holt® is a registered
trademark of Henry Holt and Company, Inc.

Published in Canada by Fitzhenry & Whiteside Ltd.,
195 Allstate Parkway, Markham, Ontario L3R 4T8.

Library of Congress Cataloging-in-Publication Data
Carrico, Mara.
Yoga journal's yoga basics: the essential beginner's guide to
yoga for a lifetime of health and fitness / Mara Carrico and the
editors of Yoga journal—with 140 photographs.—1st ed.
p.   cm.
"An Owl book."
Includes index.
ISBN 0-8050-4571-6 (alk. paper)
1. Yoga, Hatha.   I. Yoga journal.   II. Title.
RA781.7.C385   1997   97-11495
613.7'046—dc21   CIP

Henry Holt books are available for special promotions and premiums.
For details contact: Director, Special Markets.

First Edition 1997

DESIGNED BY KATE NICHOLS

Printed in the United States of America
All first editions are printed on acid-free paper. ∞

1   3   5   7   9   10   8   6   4   2

To all those seeking the clarity and compassion

that come from the yoga path

Contents

3: Styles of Hatha Yoga—A Method for Every Body *31*

PART 2:
THE PRACTICE OF YOGA

4: Breath: The Key to Health and Well-Being *43*

5: Guidelines for Practice *61*

PART 3:
COMPLETION

Acknowledgments

Writing this book has been both a challenging and a rewarding experience. Truthfully, it has been a collaborative effort and there are many to acknowledge for its completion.

First and foremost, I would like to thank Michael Gliksohn, the publisher of *Yoga Journal,* for giving me this opportunity. Secondly, I express my gratitude to Linda Sparrowe, the managing editor of *Yoga Journal,* whose guidance and many hours of restructuring and editing of my materials brought this project to the finish line. Additionally, I would like to thank Richard Miller—yoga teacher, psychologist, and friend, who mentored me throughout. Both his experience and knowledge have contributed to the substance and integrity of this work. Other *Yoga Journal* staff and contributing editors and writers who contributed significantly were Richard Leviton, Georg Feuerstein, and Anne Cushman. I thank our publisher, Henry Holt and Company, especially Bryan Oettel, who acquired the book, and senior editor Theresa Burns, who rallied it to completion. I would like to acknowledge Bill Reitzel, who provided the beautiful photographs, and models Richard Johnson, Suzanne Deason, and Linda Sparrowe, who so expertly and patiently posed for them.

Because I originally wrote this book by hand, I have many other hands to thank for its transcription onto the printed page. Preeminent among them is Georgie Salvo, for her many hours of typing and the generous use of her office. Her assistant Cheryl Ledbetter also contributed a substantial amount of time. Carolyn Avalos and Deborah Edwards provided emergency backup.

In addition to this technical assistance, I want to thank my "life support team," those who kept me going in terms of physical and mental health: Steve Paredes for chiropractic care, Kristen Lee for acupuncture and energy work, my dear friends Meg and Jim Root for emotional support, and Jackie Valdez for keeping this whole event in spiritual perspective.

I have had the pleasure and honor to have studied with many outstanding yoga teachers of a variety of methods. Although limited space precludes me listing them all, I, at the very least, wish to express my respect and gratitude for their knowledge and dedication. Among them the late Martyn Jackson, an Iyengar proponent, has most influenced the technical aspects of how I teach today. Richard Miller, who teaches in the tradition of T. K. V. Desikachar, has influenced the substance and style of my teaching.

I also wish to acknowledge all of my students and clients of this past year who have literally supported me on the physical plane and who have graciously understood when I needed to cancel classes and reschedule appointments.

Special acknowledgments go to Michael Valente and Dan Wakefield, who have encouraged me to write, and to Wilma Engel and John Engel, who were especially supportive of this particular assignment.

Finally, I'd like to take this opportunity to thank my parents, Iva May and Champ Carrico, who, in allowing me the freedom to express myself, have encouraged me on my own yoga journey.

Mara Carrico
Encinitas, California
Summer 1997

INTRODUCTION

Welcome to the World of Yoga

A couple of years ago *Yoga Journal* commissioned the Roper Poll to select a random sampling of people from all over the United States and find out what they thought about yoga. The pollsters discovered that a whopping six million Americans do yoga on a regular basis. Even better than that, sixteen million more were interested, even though they hadn't gotten around to it. We knew yoga was popular, judging from the surge in readership *Yoga Journal*'s been enjoying the last several years—and the fact that we've been around for twenty-some years—but we didn't know just how popular, or why the sudden interest.

Obviously there are many reasons people take up yoga. Some complain that their aerobic workout now creates more injuries than benefits—their knees suffer, their lower backs take a beating with every workout, or their ankles just don't absorb the impact the way they used to. Some say their doctor recommended yoga, knowing that it can help manage the increased stress in their lives. Others want something a little deeper than physical exercise, a way to combine their physical and spiritual sides. A more cynical theory suggests that the baby boomers are getting too old for the high-impact sports they used to love and are ready to embrace something gentler, kinder to their aging joints. Whatever the reason that got them into yoga, most people find that its benefits go beyond enhancing their physical health and mental acuity to promoting emotional balance and spiritual awareness as well. In short, yoga offers a way to bring balance to a person's whole being: physically, mentally, emotionally, and spiritually.

There are a lot of yoga books out there that can help. The editors at *Yoga Journal* get to see them all. We see books that focus on yoga's physical aspect, giving the reader an all-around, all-American workout. Other books tout the benefits of a particular tradition—power yoga, Iyengar yoga, or Viniyoga, for example. Still others delve into the spiritual aspects of yoga and bring us new translations of, and commentaries on, the ancient texts. But we've not seen any books that bring it all together, grounding yoga in its ancient roots and yet offering practical advice on how to integrate it into your life.

That's what we wanted to do. After all, the mission of *Yoga Journal* itself is to bring together all aspects of yoga. We don't belong to any single tradition but embrace elements of many. But for a beginning student, all these aspects can seem confusing at best, and a bit overwhelming: Do I take an Iyengar class? What about breathing—how do I do that? Do I have to believe in God to take yoga? These are questions we want to answer here. To get you started, we'll provide an overview of yoga's rich history, both in the land of its origin and in this country, bringing it up-to-date with a review of yoga's current status in today's fitness industry.

Then we'll spend the rest of the time describing the various styles of hatha practice and teaching you the fundamentals of breath, posture, relaxation, and meditation. We will then provide you with tools you can take with you as you embark on a practice of your own.

Above all, we want this book to serve as the beginning of an enjoyable and rewarding journey that will last a lifetime.

PART 1

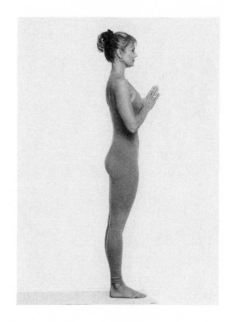

The Foundations of Yoga

1

Yoga: The Tree of Life

Although hatha yoga appears everywhere these days—at yoga centers, recreation departments, health clubs, and dance studios—yoga does not have its roots in the American physical fitness industry. In fact, scholars believe it to be more than five thousand years old, one of six orthodox philosophies evolving out of the transcendentalism of ancient India.

The Roots of Yoga

Sanskrit, the Indo-European language of the Vedas, India's ancient religious texts, gave birth to both the literature and the technique of yoga. One definition of the word Sanskrit, "well-formed, refined, perfect, or polished," connotes substance and clarity, qualities exemplified in the practice of yoga.

The Sanskrit word *yoga* has several translations and can be interpreted in many ways. It comes from the root *yug* and originally meant "to hitch up," as in attaching horses to a vehicle. Another definition was "to put to active and purposeful use." Still other translations are "yoke, join, or concentrate." Essentially, yoga has come to describe a means of uniting, or a method of discipline. A male who practices this discipline is called a *yogi,* or *yogin;* a female practitioner, a *yogini.*

Yoga comes out of an oral tradition in which the teaching was transmitted directly from teacher to student. The Indian sage Patañjali has been credited with the collation of this oral tradition into his classical work, *The Yoga Sutras*, a two-thousand-year-old treatise on yogic philosophy. A collection of one hundred ninety-five statements, the *Sutras* provide a kind of philosophical guidebook for dealing with the challenges of being human. Giving guidance on how to gain mastery over the mind and emotions and advice on spiritual growth, *The Yoga Sutras* provide the framework upon which all yoga practiced today is based. Literally meaning "thread," *sutra* has also been translated as "aphorism," which means a tersely phrased statement of truth. Another definition of *sutra* is "the condensation of the greatest amount of knowledge into the most concise description possible." Keeping these meanings in mind, we might think of the art and science of yoga as a kind of magnificent tapestry that is woven together by the threads of universal truths.

Initially, the discipline of hatha yoga—the physical aspect of yoga and the focus of this book—was developed as a vehicle for meditation. The repertoire of hatha yoga prepared the body, and particularly the nervous system, of the ancient yogis for stillness, creating the necessary physical strength and stamina that allowed the mind to remain calm.

The word *hatha* also has several translations. With *ha* meaning "sun" and *tha* meaning "moon," we have the common interpretation of hatha yoga as "a union of the pairs of opposites." A more technical translation of hatha is "force or determined effort." Thus hatha yoga, the "yoga of activity," is the yoga that addresses the body and mind and requires discipline and effort. It is the yoga that we can feel, that we can experience, right here and right now. Hatha yoga is a powerful method of self-transformation. It is the most practical of the yogas, and sages have recommended its practice in some form for millennia as preparation for all the other yogas.

The Branches of Yoga

In ancient times yoga was often referred to as a tree, a living entity with roots, a trunk, branches, blossoms, and fruit. According to the yogis, hatha yoga is one of six distinct branches; the others include *raja, karma, bhakti, jñana,* and *tantra* yoga. Each branch with its unique characteristics and function represents a particular approach to life. Some people may find one particular branch more inviting than another. However, it is important to note that involvement in one of these paths does not preclude activity in any of the others, and in fact you'll find many paths naturally overlapping.

Raja Yoga

Raja means "royal," and meditation is the focal point of this branch of yoga. This approach involves strict adherence to the eight "limbs" of yoga as outlined by Patañjali in *The Yoga Sutras.* Also found in many other branches of yoga, these limbs, or stages, follow this order: ethical standards, *yama,* self-discipline, *niyama,* posture, *asana,* breath extension or control, *pranayama,* sensory withdrawal, *pratyahara,* concentration, *dharana,* meditation, *dhyana,* and ecstasy or final liberation, *samadhi.* Raja yoga attracts individuals who are introspective and drawn to meditation. Members of religious orders and spiritual communities devote themselves to this branch of yoga. However, even though this path suggests a monastic or contemplative lifestyle, entering an ashram or monastery is not a prerequisite to practicing raja yoga.

Karma Yoga

The next branch is that of *karma* yoga or the path of service, and none of us can escape this pathway. The principle of karma yoga is that what we experience today is created by our actions in the past. Being aware of this, all of our present efforts become a way to consciously create a future that frees us from being bound by negativity and selfishness. Karma is the path of self-transcending action. We practice karma yoga whenever we perform our work and live our lives in a selfless fashion and as a way to serve others. Volunteering to serve meals in a soup kitchen or signing up for a stint with the Peace Corps or Habitat for Humanity are prime examples of the selfless service associated with the karma yoga path.

Bhakti Yoga

Bhakti yoga describes the path of devotion. Seeing the Divine in all of creation, bhakti yoga is a positive way to channel the emotions. The path of bhakti provides us with an opportunity to cultivate acceptance and tolerance for everyone we come into contact with.

Bhakti yogis express the devotional nature of their path in their every thought, word, and deed—whether they are taking out the trash or calming the anger of a loved one. Mahatma Gandhi and Martin Luther King, Jr., are prime examples of bhakti yogis. The life and work of Mother Teresa epitomize the combination of the karma and bhakti yoga paths with devotional aspects of bhakti and the selfless service of karma yoga.

Jñana Yoga

If we consider bhakti to be the yoga of the heart, then *jñana* yoga is the yoga of the mind, of wisdom, the path of the sage or scholar. This path requires development of the intellect through the study of the scriptures and texts of the yogic tradition. The jñana yoga approach is considered the most difficult and at the same time the most direct. It involves serious study and will appeal to those who are more intellectually inclined. Within the context of our Western religious traditions, Kabalistic scholars, Jesuit priests, and Benedictine monks epitomize jñana yogis.

Tantra Yoga

Finally, we have the sixth branch of the tree of yoga. Probably the most misunderstood or misinterpreted of all the yogas, *tantra* is the pathway of ritual, which includes consecrated sexuality. The key word here is "consecrated," which means to make sacred, to set apart as something holy or hallowed. In tantric practice we experience the Divine in everything we do. A reverential attitude is therefore cultivated, encouraging a ritualistic approach to life. It is amusing to note that, although tantra has become associated exclusively with sexual ritual, most tantric schools actually recommend a celibate lifestyle. In essence, tantra is the most esoteric of the six major branches. It will appeal to those yogis who enjoy ceremony and relate to the feminine principle of the cosmos, which yogis call *shakti.* If you see—and are deeply moved by—the significance behind celebration and ritual (holidays, birthdays, anniversaries, and other rites of passage), tantra yoga may be for you. Many tantric yogis find magic in all types of ceremony, whether it be a Japanese tea ceremony, the consecration of the Eucharist in a Catholic mass, or the consummation of a relationship.

Combining the Paths

You may already be involved in one or more of these branches. For example, you may already be a hatha yogi—or yogini—practicing the postures with a teacher or by yourself. If you are a hospice volunteer for AIDS patients, or a participant in a Big Brother/Big Sister program, you are actively practicing karma yoga. Perhaps reading this book will spark an in-depth study of yoga philosophy, setting you on the path of jñana yoga. Remember you need not be limited to one expression— you may practice hatha yoga, taking care of your physical body, while simultaneously cultivating the lifestyle of a bhakti yogi, expressing your compassion for everyone you meet. Trust that whichever avenue of yogic expression draws your interest, it will probably be the right yoga path for you.

To further your understanding of these pathways of yogic expression, let's take a closer look at the aforementioned eight limbs of yoga.

The Limbs of Yoga

In *The Yoga Sutras* of Patañjali, the eightfold path is called *ashtanga,* which literally means "eight limbs" (*ashta* = eight, *anga* = limb). These eight steps basically act as guidelines on how to live a meaningful and purposeful life. They serve as a prescription for moral and ethical conduct and self-discipline; they direct attention toward one's health; and they help us to acknowledge the spiritual aspects of our nature.

Yama

The first limb, *yama,* deals with one's ethical standards and sense of integrity, focusing on our behavior and how we conduct ourselves in life. These are universal practices that relate best to what we know as the Golden Rule, "Do unto others as you would have them do unto you." The five yamas are

> *Ahimsa:* non-violence or non-injury
> *Satya:* truthfulness
> *Asteya:* non-stealing
> *Brahmacharya:* continence
> *Aparigraha:* non-covetousness

Niyama

Niyama, the second limb, are individual practices having to do with self-discipline and spiritual observances. Regularly attending temple or church services, saying grace before meals, developing your own personal meditation practice, or making a habit of taking contemplative walks alone would all come under this heading. The five niyamas are

Saucha: cleanliness
Santosa: contentment
Tapas: heat; spiritual austerities
Svadhyaya: study of the sacred scriptures and of one's self
Isvara pranidhana: surrender to God

Asana

Asana, the postures practiced in yoga, comprise the third limb. In the yogic view, the body is a temple of spirit, the care of which is an important stage of our spiritual growth. Through the practice of asana, we develop the habit of discipline and the ability to concentrate, both of which are necessary for meditation.

Pranayama

Generally translated as breath control, this fourth stage consists of techniques designed to gain mastery over the respiratory process while recognizing the connection between the breath, the mind, and the emotions. As implied by the literal translation of *pranayama,* "life force extension," yogis believe that it not only rejuvenates the body but actually extends life itself. You can practice pranayama as an isolated technique (i.e., simply sitting and performing a number of breathing exercises), or integrate it into your daily hatha yoga routine.

These first four stages of Patañjali's ashtanga yoga concentrate on refining our personalities, gaining mastery over the body, and developing an energetic awareness of ourselves, all of which prepares us for the second half of this journey, which deals with the senses, the mind, and attaining a higher state of consciousness.

Pratyahara

Pratyahara, the fifth limb, means withdrawal or sensory transcendence. It is during this stage that we make the conscious effort to draw our awareness away from the external world and outside stimuli. Keenly aware of, yet cultivating a detachment from, our senses, we direct our attention internally. The practice of pratyahara provides us with an opportunity to step back and take a look at ourselves. This withdrawal allows us to objectively observe our cravings: habits that are perhaps detrimental to our health and which likely interfere with our inner growth.

Dharana

As each stage prepares us for the next, the practice of pratyahara creates the setting for *dharana,* or concentration. Having relieved ourselves of outside distractions, we can now deal with the distractions of the mind itself. No easy task! In the practice of concentration, which precedes meditation, we learn how to slow down the thinking process by concentrating on a single mental object: a specific energetic center in the body, an image of a deity, or the silent repetition of a sound. We, of course, have already begun to develop our powers of concentration in the previous three stages of posture, breath control, and withdrawal of the senses. In asana and pranayama, although we pay attention to our actions, our attention travels. Our focus constantly shifts as we fine-tune the many nuances of any particular posture or breathing technique. In pratyahara we become self-observant; now, in dharana, we focus our attention on a single point. Extended periods of concentration naturally lead to meditation.

Dhyana

Meditation or contemplation, the seventh stage of ashtanga, is the uninterrupted flow of concentration. Although concentration (*dharana*) and meditation (*dhyana*) may appear to be one and the same, a fine line of distinction exists between these two stages. Where dharana practices one-pointed attention, dhyana is ultimately a state of being keenly aware without focus. At this stage, the mind has been quieted, and in the stillness it produces few or no thoughts at all. The strength and stamina it takes to reach this state of stillness is quite impressive. But don't give up. While this may seem a difficult, if not impossible, task, remember that yoga is a process. Even though we may not attain the "picture perfect" pose, or the ideal state of consciousness, we surely benefit at every stage of our progress.

Samadhi

Patañjali describes this eighth and final stage of ashtanga as a state of ecstasy. At this stage, the meditator merges with his or her point of focus and transcends the self altogether. The meditator comes to realize a profound connection to the Divine, an interconnectedness with all living things. With this realization comes the "peace that passeth all understanding"; the experience of bliss and being at one with the Universe. On the surface, this may seem to be a rather lofty, "holier than thou" kind of goal. However, if we pause to examine what we really want to get out of life, would not joy, fulfillment, and freedom somehow find their way onto our list of hopes, wishes, and desires? What Patañjali has described as the completion of the yogic path is what, deep down, all human beings aspire to: peace. We also might give some thought to the fact that this ultimate stage of yoga— enlightenment—can neither be bought nor possessed. It can only be experienced, the price of which is the continual devotion of the aspirant.

Yoga Comes to America

Although hatha yoga—the third of Patañjali's eight-limbed path—eventually became the yoga of choice for most Americans, it was the more contemplative stages—raja and jñana yoga—that initially ignited the interest of an exclusive group of Americans over one hundred fifty years ago. Referred to as transcendentalists themselves and part of an elite group of intellectuals known as the Concord Circle, Ralph Waldo Emerson and Henry David Thoreau drew inspiration from the *Bhagavad Gita*. This sacred Hindu text, written in the form of a philosophical dialogue, is an integral part of yoga's literary heritage. And so it was that these men, two of America's most influential poet/philosophers of that era, in Concord, Massachusetts, planted the seeds for the growth of yoga in America.

Representing only a small segment of our culture at that time, those inspired by Emerson and Thoreau's enthusiasm for this "exotic" foreign philosophy kept the interest alive. Bronson Alcott and William Henry Channing, also members of the Concord Circle, saw to it that Edwin Arnold found an American publisher for his biography of Gautama Buddha, *The Light in Asia,* in 1879. Only four years earlier, Colonel Henry Steel Olcott, a prominent New York lawyer, and Helene Blavatsky, a Russian émigré and occultist, established the Theosophical Society, in New York City. Blavatsky, as renowned for being a cigar-smoking eccentric as she was for her esoteric knowledge, went on to publish *Isis Unveiled* in 1877 and *The Secret Doctrine* in 1888. These two voluminous treatises collectively divulged many of the secret teachings of the ancient Vedic texts.

By 1893, the stage had been appropriately set for the arrival of Swami Vivekananda at the World Parliament of Religions, which took place in Chicago, Illinois. Speaking to a largely American audience, Vivekananda lectured on the merits of raja yoga, a theme he would reiterate often during his two-year stay in the United States. In 1899 he returned again to America where he founded the New York Vedanta Society, a thriving community that continues to focus on four of the six branches of yoga: raja, karma, bhakti, and jñana.

The yoga of the swamis who followed Vivekananda to America was mostly philosophical in nature, with nominal attention paid to the practice of hatha yoga. It took several decades for the physical aspect of this philosophy to really take hold. But, in the interim, Yogendra Mastamani, landing in Long Island in 1919, began to demonstrate the power of hatha yoga to Northeastern America. His own guru, Paramahansa Madhavadasaji, initiated a growing movement in early twentieth-century India to establish hatha yoga as a viable physical culture. Madhavadasaji encouraged another one of his students, Kuvalayananda, to create the Kaivalyadhama Ashram and Research Institute near Pune, India, where physicians and scientists could explore the more scientific aspects of asana practice. Before Mastamani left the United States in 1922, he founded the first American branch of Kaivalyadhama and began a dialogue with the American medical community, particularly the alternative physicians of the time, establishing yoga as a viable healing therapy. His connection with Benedict Lust, the founder of naturopathy, began a relationship between yoga and alternative medicine and healing practices that continues today.

Another outstanding contributor to the growth of yoga in America, Paramahansa Yogananda, came to Boston in 1920 where he addressed the International Congress of Religious Liberals. After a three-year tenure in Boston, Yogananda toured the United States and, in 1925, wound up in Los Angeles where he founded the Self Realization Fellowship (SRF). SRF has attracted hundreds of thousands of followers throughout the years and remains a strong force within the yoga community. Yogananda's *Autobiography of a Yogi,* penned in 1946, six years before his death, turned an entire generation of seekers on to yoga and Eastern spirituality and continues to inspire people today.

It took the efforts of another Russian woman to solidify the position of the physical aspect of yoga within our culture. Indra Devi, known as the "First Lady of Yoga" in America, set down roots in Hollywood, California, and opened her first U.S. yoga studio in 1947. Born in Riga, Latvia, in 1899, Indra Devi (or Mataji as she is known) spent several years in India prior to coming west, studying with Krishnamacharya, a man many consider to be the father of modern-day hatha yoga, and teaching classes. Hollywood luminaries quickly embraced her teachings, and such stars as Jennifer Jones, Gloria Swanson, and Robert Ryan helped bring the public's attention to the benefits of yoga. But Mataji's influence went far beyond the entertainment industry. Credited with almost single-handedly establishing a niche for American hatha yoga, she taught thousands of students and trained hundreds of teachers.

After leaving Hollywood, Mataji established a yoga center in Tecate, Mexico. She has since settled in Buenos Aires, Argentina, where she continues to teach and practice. She often returns to India which she considers her true spiritual home. In addition to her great contribution to the American yoga scene, Indra Devi remains a guiding force in yoga throughout the world.

While Yogananda and Indra Devi relied on their classes, lectures, and books to reach thousands of aspiring yogis, the medium of television provided a venue through which millions more could learn this ancient discipline. Beginning with Richard Hittleman in 1961 and followed by Lilias Folan nearly a decade later, Americans began practicing yoga in front of their TV sets in droves. Hittleman, who sadly passed away in 1991, wrote, among his many other books, *The Twenty-Eight-Day Yoga Plan,* which sold millions of copies. Lilias continues to be a spokesperson for the American yoga community through her many videos, television programs, and personal appearances.

As middle America was tuning in to Hittleman and Lilias, a whole other segment of the population was turning on to the benefits of deep breathing. The social and political climate of the sixties and seventies created a free-spirited individualism that encouraged people of all ages to question and explore their values, both materially and spiritually. This exploration led to an intense interest in Asian cultures and exotic philosophies. Fueled by the Beatles' much publicized visit to India and their initiation into Maharishi Mahesh Yogi's Transcendental

Meditation—along with the publication of Ram Dass's *Be Here Now*—meditation became the order of the day.

In response to the growing need for spiritual awakening, gurus—both foreign and domestic—sprung up all over America, and whole communities were established along with them. These environments provided the space and supportive atmosphere in which one could live and work while pursuing the study and practice of yoga. One such community, the Ananda Village, a 750-acre spread in Nevada City, California, was founded in 1968 by Swami Kriyananda, an American disciple of Paramahansa Yogananda. The nearly three hundred fifty residents practice Yogananda's kriya yoga system, a combination of pranayama and asana that stimulates the more subtle currents of energy in the body. The community offers schooling for its resident children through eighth grade. Many of the adult residents are employed both on and off the property in several private and Ananda-owned businesses.

By the end of the 1970s, several spiritual communities were thriving. Baba Hari Dass founded Mt. Madonna near Santa Cruz, California, and Swami Satchidananda's Yogaville established roots in Buckingham, Virginia. Today many residential and nonresidential communities exist to bring the teachings of their particular spiritual lineage to the masses. Whether they espouse Hindu, Buddhist, or Taoist philosophy, these centers promote a simple and healthy lifestyle.

The more physical aspect of yoga—hatha yoga—also began to evolve during this time, with the arrival of several visiting teachers from India. Yogi Bhajan, B. K. S. Iyengar, and Swami Vishnu-devananda all made an indelible mark on the landscape of American yoga, each bringing a distinct style of hatha yoga to the attention of eager students. Each of these styles, along with several others, will be outlined in greater detail in chapter 3.

Yoga and American Fitness

By the 1970s, Americans were fast becoming obsessed with looking good and keeping fit: the quicker the better. While yoga may have been a nice adjunct for some, it didn't shed unwanted pounds or trim those thighs fast enough for most people. They turned to aerobic exercise—"no pain, no gain"—in a big way, and the fitness industry soon evolved into a multibillion-dollar business. Much of this obsession can be traced back to the research of Dr. Kenneth Cooper, a major in the

U.S. Air Force, who by 1968 had conducted studies on the exercise regimens and fitness levels of more than five thousand subjects. Finding that those regimens that promoted aerobic exercise clearly achieved the best results, he published his findings in his best-selling book, *Aerobics*. Based on a point system, Cooper ranked exercises solely by the benefit they had on the cardiovascular system: running came in first, followed by swimming, cycling, and walking.

Taking this information about "aerobic points" to heart, a young Air Force wife, Jackie Sorenson, began practicing her teaching and dance skills on a group of officers' wives in 1969. Using movement and music to create the training effect Cooper prescribed in his book, Sorenson and her husband formed Aerobic Dancing, Inc., in 1970. Two years later another high-energy dancer, Judi Sheppard Missett, created Jazzercise, promoting dance choreographed for the nondancer as a way to get and stay fit.

Meanwhile, with more than twenty million Americans participating in aerobics by 1980, the number of injuries reported was staggering. Studies showed that 75 percent of aerobics instructors and 45 percent of participants sustained some type of injury. Hearts may have been getting healthier, but muscles, ligaments, and joints were being destroyed. The combination of overtraining, focus on high-impact aerobics, poor body mechanics, and above all lack of good instructor training threatened the very activity that had initially been created to promote health and longevity.

Still, the fitness industry was loath to abandon what it saw as the benefits of aerobic exercise, and it continued to view yoga as something much too esoteric for the masses. Instead it focused on establishing industry standards which would ensure safety and quality instruction for aerobics teachers. Certification programs, conferences, and workshops were developed—and still exist today—thanks to the efforts of IDEA (International Association of Fitness Professionals) and the American Council on Exercise. In the beginning these industry watchdogs were extremely conservative, designing guidelines and recommending exercise techniques purely for the aerobic dance instructor, still buying into the theory that a healthy heart was the only indicator of a healthy body.

Today, mostly due to its own research efforts, the industry has taken a 180-degree about-face in its relationship to yoga. Although it still embraces cardiovascular conditioning as the main focus in most of its programs, it now agrees that strength and flexibility are necessary components of a complete fitness package and that stress management is essential to maintaining good health.

Walking has replaced running as the aerobic exercise that exercise physiologists most often recommend, and feeling better now takes precedence over looking better. "Listen to your body, go at your own pace" has replaced "no pain, no gain" and "go for the burn" as the fitness mantra, and as a result, hatha yoga has taken its rightful place as a viable way of keeping the body—and the mind—healthy and strong.

Of course it didn't hurt that the perennial queen of the fitness video market, Jane Fonda herself, publicly embraced yoga. The release of her 1994 *Yoga Exercise Workout* marked a whole new shift in the industry toward a more contemplative approach to working out. Other celebrities got on the bandwagon with their own videos, and even the shoe companies unwittingly lent their support. The Reebok Flexible Strength Program, developed by physical therapist and yoga enthusiast Deborah Ellison as part of Reebok's instructor training programs, includes a substantial number of yoga postures. What all this signifies is that hatha yoga has, at long last, found the respect and recognition it always deserved from the fitness industry. Yoga is now standard fare in the programs of gyms, health clubs, YW and YMCAs, and recreation centers everywhere. In fact, from your local gym to the most exclusive health spa, yoga is likely to be one of the most popular items on the fitness schedule.

The Mind-Body Movement

Yoga's popularity in today's fitness field signals a whole new trend in how we view exercise. It also represents the creation of a specific category in the industry called Mind-Body Fitness or Mind-Body Exercise. Reflecting the recognition and application of the mind-body connection that has evolved in health care, the mind-body fitness arena is expanding at an impressive rate.

Defined by IDEA's Mind-Body Fitness Committee as "physical exercise executed with a profound inwardly directed awareness or focus," mind-body exercise encompasses a number of modalities ranging from centuries-old disciplines to modern-day adaptations of these traditional forms.

Obviously, the mind always plays a part in directing the body, regardless of the nature of the activity, whether it be Western or Eastern, vigorous or gentle, aerobically oriented or not; however, there are several factors that qualify an exercise to be mind-body specific. In addition to internally directed focus, the most common characteristics of mind-body exercise are:

- It is often performed at a slower pace than other exercise;
- It emphasizes quality, rather than quantity, of movement;
- Its activities are process-focused rather than goal-oriented and are performed in a noncompetitive spirit;
- It emphasizes listening to your body and learning to pay attention to your feelings.

Mind-body activities have tangible benefits that complement or equal the benefits of conventional exercise. A contemplative state of being is naturally created that is not dissimilar to the alpha state or slowing of the brain waves which takes place in the beginning stages of a meditation practice. What happens in mind-body fitness is the development of what is called your proprioceptive cognition, the tangible knowledge of your physical self and your movement in space. With the development of this inner awareness, you become more receptive to the processes that are taking place in your body right now. In other words, as you become present to what is going on, you can become more objective about or detached from the outcome. What matters is the experience, not the result.

In mind-body exercise, the benefits are the positive by-products of the internally directed attention you give yourself. For example, increased self-confidence and a sense of inner peace are just two of the barometers of progress in mind-body exercise. So, rather than taking your heart rate several times during class or measuring body fat, you might ask yourself the following questions:

- Is my level of energy high or low?
- Is the quality of that energy positive or negative?
- Am I feeling calm and centered or agitated and scattered?
- Where in my body do I feel tension, stress, discomfort, or fatigue?
- How is my breathing—long or short, even or erratic?

As you can see, mind-body fitness is very Eastern both in character and in approach. While the various styles of hatha yoga and the different forms of martial arts, especially chi kung, head the list of mind-body exercise techniques, others include the Alexander Technique, the Feldenkrais Method, and an exercise system based on the work of Joseph Pilates, the latter three dating back to the beginning of this century.

Many other exercise modalities have come along, especially within the last thirty years, which are also considered mind-body. Some of them are more artistic in nature, having been developed by dancers, such as the work of Bonnie Bainbridge Cohen and Emilie Conrad-Da'oud. Others have come out of the fitness arena itself, such as the work of Debbie and Carlos Rosas, who created NIA, neuromuscular integrative action, a form of aerobic dance.

As more exercise enthusiasts are attracted to the realm of mind-body fitness for whatever reason, whether it's because their doctor recommended it or because it just feels better, this arena of the industry has proven to be a viable and beneficial option for everyone. And, ironically, the impetus behind this relatively modern phenomenon is a centuries-old practice called hatha yoga.

2

Hatha Yoga—More than Just a Stretch

Whereas yoga and its principles of posture, movement, and breath fit neatly into the mind-body fitness category, hatha yoga is more than a mere stretching routine that incorporates breathing exercises—it represents the development of a unique physical culture which has long recognized that posture, movement, and breath are inextricably connected to mental equanimity. This physical culture has evolved over the centuries as a way of preparing the body for meditation. Creating an elaborate methodology to bring about optimal functioning of the entire system, hatha yoga addresses the human being on a psychological as well as physiological level. All the systems of the body are affected: muscular, skeletal, circulatory, respiratory, digestive, reproductive, endocrine, lymphatic, and nervous. A psychophysical element also exists within hatha yoga—the idea that posture, movement, and breath affect the emotions as well as the mind.

Within the tradition of yoga, hatha yoga has its own distinct heritage, a heritage entwined within a mythology that, while offering us little factual information, is rich in symbolism. Many of these myths are about yogis and deities who possessed extraordinary supernatural powers and demonstrated great psychic abilities.

Although quite a few manuscripts survive that represent the more pragmatic elements of this discipline, very few provide useful descriptions or technical step-by-step instructions for the postures themselves. Instead, the practice of hatha yoga has endured through oral transmission by a lineage of teachers who have served as links in this chain of knowledge. This lineage officially dates back to the eleventh century, when the philosophy of hatha yoga was first articulated by Goraksha (or Goraknath), considered to be the founding father of hatha yoga. Examples of texts attributed to him still exist. While Goraksha himself may have been only a symbolic character, the body of knowledge allegedly recorded by him has served as a foundation for the evolution of hatha yoga.

The Union of Opposites

Literally translated, *hatha* means "force," "power," or "effort." Thus, we have the powerful yoga—the yoga that develops strength and determination in order to unify the body and mind. Additionally, the commonly accepted translations of *ha* as "sun" and *tha* as "moon" reflect the conceptual basis of the practice itself: that of opening up the body as a vehicle for *Prana*—the vital energy of life—while bringing harmony to the whole system.

The two opposing aspects of this vital energy can be viewed as expansion and contraction, *prana* and *apana* (which you'll learn about later on), or *brhmana* and *langhana,* Sanskrit for "expanding" and "fasting," respectively. These opposing energies reside in all the postures and in the breath itself. Through the application of hatha yoga techniques, these aspects are brought into balance. In fact, a vast repertoire has developed toward accomplishing this balance. This repertoire consists of postures and movements, *asanas,* as well as breathing, *pranayama,* and relaxation techniques, all of which are designed as either active or passive, requiring effort or relaxation, to work together to bring about optimal health and well-being. This energetic duality is represented throughout hatha yoga by the technical principles governing the practice itself: expansion and contraction, pose and counterpose, dynamic and static, and steady and comfortable.

Expansion/Contraction

Brhmana, the expanding aspect of vital energy, is reflected in the inhalation and retention of the breath. Brhmana is associated with the creation of heat and light and invigorates the whole person. The energy you receive from this aspect is stimulating, extroverted, and active. The postures which promote this expansive quality are backbends—poses that hyperextend or arch the spine and open up the chest.

Langhana, the fasting or contracting principle, connects to the exhalation and suspension of the breath at the end of the exhalation. Langhana energy is cold and dark, relaxing and pacifying, creating feelings of introspection and calm. Postures which promote this contracting principle include forward bends and twisting poses.

Pose/Counterpose

The aspects of expansion and contraction are carried through the entire structure of your practice in the form of pose and counterpose. The application of this principle ensures that the spine and the musculature can actively be brought into balance. Backbends follow forward bends (and vice versa), side-stretching poses and twists happen on both sides. Yoga also expresses this principle energetically: A series of seated poses which are passive follow standing postures which are more active.

Dynamic/Static

This principle relates to the approach we take in any given posture. In this context, dynamic denotes expansion through repetitive motion—moving into and out of a specific posture, perhaps several times, before holding the pose itself in a static fashion. Moving into and out of a posture first warms up the muscles and prepares the joints to take on the demands required to hold the pose.

It is interesting to note how this principle plays upon itself. We need to have a certain amount of stillness in our movements in order to remain balanced and centered as we go into and out of a posture. Conversely, within the stillness of holding a posture, we must continue to be aware of movement on a more subtle plane—the movement of the breath within the body, for example, and the delicate adjustments taking place in the spine and in the musculature as we hold the pose.

Steady/Comfortable

Within this framework of dualities is yet another principle—that of being steady or firm, yet comfortable, in all of our postures. In Sanskrit these two qualities are referred to as *sthira* and *sukha.* Patañjali, in *The Yoga Sutras,* clearly states that these two qualities must be present in any given asana, or you are not truly practicing yoga. *Sthira* means to be alert as well as steady and firm—the opposite of being unstable, unconscious, or flaccid. In addition to comfort, *sukha* denotes joy, pleasure, and ease—the opposite of *dukha* which means pain or suffering.

Maintaining steadiness and comfort is an especially important principle—no matter how simple or challenging a posture may be—as it helps us monitor our efforts, keep us focused on what we're doing, and ensure the safety of our practice.

Note that ease or comfort, *sukha,* never implies easy—as in "nothing to it." What it does mean is that we seek equanimity in each pose. At the same time, however, we want to be conscious—alert and stable, *sthira,* on the lookout for any pain or discomfort that we might be experiencing. This concept will teach you to listen to your body: If there is pain, you need to pay attention to it and adjust your efforts accordingly. This doesn't mean that you just do whatever's easiest for you. You need challenge, and at times you will experience degrees of *reasonable intensity* within the postures. For instance, if your hamstrings are tight, of course you'll feel them when you do a forward bend. However, if you remain focused and alert, keeping the body and breath steady, you will be able to maintain the pose with a degree of comfort and ease. On the other hand, if your muscles are shaking and your breathing feels unsteady, your body is telling you that you have gone beyond your current capability and you're on your way to pain, soreness, or pulled muscles—in essence, *dukha.*

As you can see, hatha yoga is actually a highly evolved and sophisticated approach to fitness and health. Despite this complexity, however, it is important to remember that the basis of this method is simple and perpetual—creating balance. This theme will be evident in every aspect of the practice. Bearing this in mind will keep you grounded in terms of purpose and enhance the satisfaction you experience at every stage of your progress.

The Structure of a Yoga Class

It's all well and good to learn the fundamentals of creating balance in yoga, but what does that mean exactly as you get ready to embark on a practice of your own? Let's take a look at how the fundamentals of duality—the physical, *asana,* and the energetic, *pranayama,* expansion and contraction, pose and counterpose—appear in an actual yoga class to create balance and well-being.

Yoga Postures (*Asanas*)

Although the term *asana* has come to mean pose, posture, or position, it original-ly meant a seat—the place or material on which the yogi sat to meditate. It also meant "to sit" or "to be seated." This original meaning of *asana* lends a deeper sig-nificance to the practice: The postures are *sit*uations providing us with the oppor-tunity to create poise and equanimity.

The postures themselves fall into the following categories: standing, seated, supine (lying on the back), prone (lying face down), and inversions (such as Headstand, Shoulderstand, or Elbowstand). Within this framework, the spine moves through its full range of motion—forward bends (forward flexion), back-bends (hyperextension), twists (rotation of spine), and side bends (lateral flexion). Yogic postures give continual attention to spinal extension (extending or length-ening), whether you are in a static, neutral position or moving your spine in any given direction. The intent of proper practice is to create a balance of strength and flexibility in the entire musculo-skeletal system. An element of stamina comes into play as well, as we develop the ability to sustain the postures.

Essentially, asana practice provides us with a three-step system: creating the flexibility to get into a posture, building the strength to hold the pose in proper alignment, and developing the stamina to maintain it for longer durations. The last step—that of stamina—requires concentration and an opportunity to focus on the breath.

In addition to affecting the musculo-skeletal system, the postures enhance the whole of internal function. All of the postures increase circulation throughout the body, while affecting both the respiratory and nervous systems. Other systems of the body, as well as the organs, also benefit from yoga poses in very specific ways, depending upon which poses you choose, how you position your body, the pace you set, and how you breathe during practice.

Bringing the systems and organs of the body into balance has a profound influ-ence on the psyche as well. This acknowledgment is based on the mind-body premise that emotional stability and calmness of mind reflect balance brought about in the physical body. Specific postures in combination with prescribed breathing patterns can either stimulate (creating an energetic and outgoing demeanor) or pacify (encouraging contemplation and a more introverted or passive state of being).

Breath (*Pranayama*)

The breath represents much more than the oxygen we take into our lungs. Even though hatha yoga incorporates specific breathing techniques to enhance the effects of the postures, *pranayama,* or breath extension, is a category unto itself.

Ayama means "extension." *Prana* has several connotations—breath, respiration, life, vitality, wind, energy, strength, spirit, and soul. By acknowledging all of these meanings, we are dealing with much more than oxygen when we "extend the breath." Another definition uses *yama* meaning "control" instead of *ayama,* hence the popular translation "breath control." While asana and pranayama contain both physical and psychological benefits, pranayama also represents a subtle, energetic level of awareness.

Pranayama exercises begin simply, progressively demanding greater refinement of the breath. At the beginning stages, pranayama involves slowing down the pace of the breath and breathing rhythmically—making the inhalations and exhalations even in length. Gradually, you learn more complicated exercises, such as the alternate nostril breath (breathing in and out of only one nostril at a time, while closing off the other nostril with the fingers), breath retentions (holding the breath in after the inhalation), and breath suspensions (holding the breath out after exhalation).

The benefits of pranayama practice abound, with the obvious—improving the respiratory system—topping the list. Technically, increasing oxygen intake enhances functioning of the entire system. Your posture will automatically improve, since breathing correctly means aligning the spine properly and consciously engaging the musculature of the torso. Once again, as in asana practice, a yogi may articulate the breath to create specific results: Emphasis placed on inhalation will generally create a stimulating or energizing effect on the system; when a more passive or relaxed state is desired, exhalation is usually emphasized.

Types of Yoga Poses

The structure of most hatha yoga classes incorporates poses designed to balance the body and the mind, generally including as many active, expanding postures, *brhmana,* as passive, contracting ones, *langhana.* The following gives you a brief introduction to the types of postures you would practice in most yoga classes.

Standing Postures. The strength and longevity of any structure—even the human form—depends upon its foundation. Standing poses help us build a physical foundation of strength and stability, offering an excellent way to get grounded and centered "by standing on your own two feet." The list of standing postures is long and includes many one-leg balances that are especially challenging and demand concentration. On a psychological level, standing poses create confidence, enhance willpower, and strengthen character. (Figure 1.)

Seated Postures. Reflecting the original meaning of *asana,* "the seat on which the yogi sits to meditate," seated postures have a more contemplative flavor. A number of the static seated poses are designed for pranayama and meditation practice, but there are also quite a few seated forward bends which require flexibility in the lower back and entail stretching the hamstrings. Twisted seated poses offer many benefits. The twisting or torsion of the spine often encourages a natural adjustment of the vertebrae which, since major nerves run along the spine, stimulates the nervous system. This torsion from a twisted posture (i.e., thigh drawn

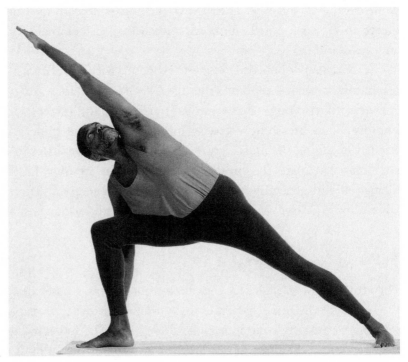

FIG. 1

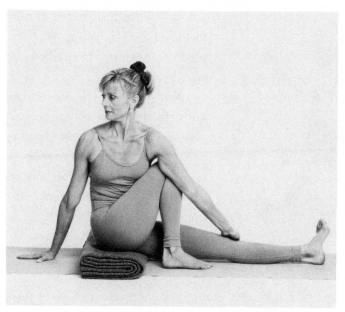

FIG. 2

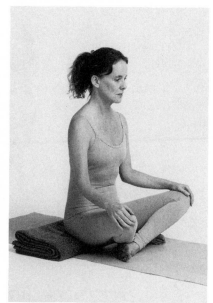

FIG. 3

up and crossing the chest) compresses the organs of digestion, enhancing elimination. (Figure 2.)

Although seated postures may look meditative, for many of us they can be quite challenging. The tight hips and weak lower backs encouraged by our "chair society" make sitting on the floor yoga-style much less serene than intended! Solution: Use a folded blanket or flat cushion under your hips. (Figure 3.) (See The Use of Props.) On the other hand, seated postures give us the most pronounced feedback on our progress. As you begin to feel more comfortable sitting on the floor, you'll know that you have created more flexibility in your hips and strength in your back.

Prone Postures (facing the floor, either on hands and knees or on your stomach). These postures are more active, as they include either weight-bearing poses or backbends. Prone postures are especially strengthening for the arms and the musculature of the back. The weight-bearing postures require a certain flexibility of the shoulder joints, as well as strength in the wrists. The back-bending poses require and build abdominal strength. Back-care specialists using the "McKenzie method" of physical therapy will often employ many of these prone postures, so

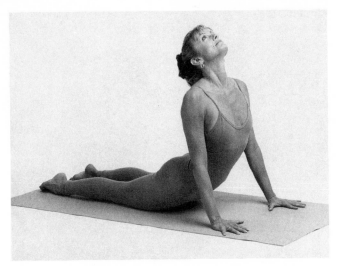

FIG. 4

you may have seen moves similar to Cobra Pose if you've ever had physical therapy prescribed for your back. (Figure 4.)

Note that there are several postures done on your knees. If you have knee problems, you may need to skip these active poses or use a chair for support. Sometimes a folded towel or extra padding under the knees works well, or even athletic knee pads. (See The Use of Props.)

Supine Postures (lying on the back). An immediate energetic shift takes place when we turn over onto our backs. We can shift gears as the body and mind receive the message that we are in preparation for relaxation or sleep. Although some challenging postures may be performed from the supine position (i.e., back-bends and postures involving abdominal strength), the context will be more passive.

Some of the supine postures are especially beneficial to the spine and are considered remedial for the back. Knee-to-Chest Pose and the pelvic tilt, which begins the Two-Legged Platform, are not dissimilar to the movements in the classic "Williams' Flexion" series, often prescribed by back specialists and physical therapists for lower back discomfort. (Figure 5A.)

The floor may also be considered a prop. Lying on the floor allows you to feel your back on a surface that is flat. This can be a handy reference for alignment and symmetry.

Inversions. Reversing the body's relationship to gravity has many benefits: It increases circulation, stimulates the brain, and enhances the glandular system. Although they are not recommended during menstruation, inversions such as Headstand, Shoulderstand, and Plough are so beneficial that they're often referred to as the King, Queen, and Prince of asanas. (Figure 5B.)

FIG. 5B

FIG. 5A

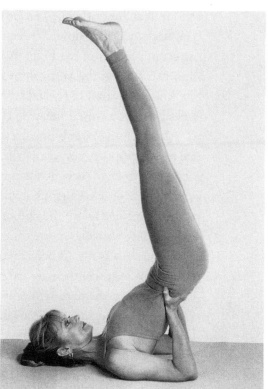

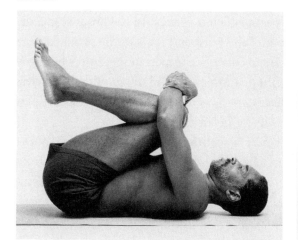

The Mechanics of Yoga Practice

In order to practice effectively, you need to have a working knowledge of the fundamental principles of posture, movement, and breath. The following information will help you understand the mechanics involved in aligning the spine, moving efficiently, and breathing correctly. These rules will provide you with a formula you can refer to, whether you practice at home or participate in a class. Although on occasion there may be exceptions, for the most part these basic rules will serve you well, no matter what style of yoga you choose or what your level of accomplishment is.

Posture and the Alignment of Your Spine

When we talk about good posture, we are referring to the alignment of the spine and the placement of the limbs within the poses or asanas themselves. Whether you are standing on your feet or on your head, sitting in a chair or on the floor, lying face up or face down, we can still trace what's called the "plumb line," or the correct alignment of the body. When you're standing up, this plumb line (as seen from the side) is the vertical and congruent alignment of the earlobe, shoulder, hip, knee, and front of the ankle. When sitting in a chair or on the floor with your knees bent, you would measure the plumb line from the earlobe to the hip.

Although the plumb line itself is a straight one, the spine will have its own natural and appropriate curves. At the neck is the cervical curve, which is concave. Then comes the thoracic curve at the upper back, which is convex. In the lower spine, the concave lumbar curve begins at the back of the waist and leads to the sacral curve, a convex shape just above the tailbone. These curves are important because when they are in balance with one another they facilitate movement, and the spine deflects stress or weight more easily. When any of these curves becomes exaggerated, another part of the spine must compensate, often resulting in back problems.

Changes in the natural alignment may be subtle, with little or minimal negative effect on posture and movement. However, more dramatic deviations, from injury, disease, or poor posture, will create more exaggerated effects on the symmetry of the body and will likely produce a chronic state of discomfort. Of course, we need to pay attention to this signal of discomfort and seek the advice of a health professional, back specialist, chiropractor, or physical therapist. In other words, the practice of asanas alone is not designed to cure severe cases of spinal misalignment or chronic pain. If you do suffer from back problems, confer with your doctor or health specialist before starting a yoga practice.

If, on the other hand, you have a history of poor posture or suffer from mild deviations of the spine, a balanced practice of asanas may help you by bringing your attention to the imbalances in your structure and habits—how you sit, walk, stand, and sleep—or by alleviating the stress that may be causing or exacerbating pain or tightness.

Common Deviations of the Spine

The following is a list of the most common deviations in spinal alignment, their possible causes, and ways in which yoga can help. Keep in mind that every body is unique and that these general recommendations refer only to the poses and exercises outlined in this book. For a more individualized routine, consult a yoga therapist—a teacher who specializes in remedial programs for various disorders.

Lordosis. This condition—commonly called a sway back—refers to an exaggerated curvature in the lower back or lumbar region of the spine. Lordosis often develops due to a weakness in the abdominals and a corresponding tightness in the hip flexors—the front of the hips and thighs.

FOCUS ON: Lengthening the lower back, strengthening the abdominals, and stretching the hip flexors.

POSES THAT MAY HELP: For the back: Dvipada Pitham (Two-Legged Platform), Apanasana (Knee-to-Chest Pose), and the preparatory stages of Jathara Parivartanasana (Twisted Stomach Pose) or Paripurna Navasana (Full Boat Pose).

For the hip flexors: Heel-to-Buttock One-Leg Balance Pose; the lunge position of the Sun Salute.

Kyphosis. Often referred to as "dowager's hump," this is an exaggerated curve in the upper back or thoracic area of the spine. Indicative of weak upper back muscles and tight chest muscles, this condition is usually accompanied by a poor respiratory system.

FOCUS ON: Rolling the shoulders back and down, opening the chest, and strengthening the upper back. Kyphosis can often severely restrict the shoulder joints; therefore it's also helpful to practice a number of the basic shoulder joint openers and range of motion movements.

POSES THAT MAY HELP: For opening the chest and strengthening the back, practice Cobra Pose and its variations, including Standing Cobra and modified Downward-Facing Dog at the wall. To open the shoulder joints and improve range of motion, practice Basic Supine with arms resting on the floor, above the head, with elbows slightly bent; or from a standing position, bring your arms up and out to the sides at shoulder level, and practice turning the palms up and down, rotating the arms from within the shoulder joints without collapsing the chest.

Scoliosis. A lateral curve or deviation in the alignment of the spine, scoliosis shows up as a pronounced asymmetry in the back muscles (i.e., one side is more developed than the other). The pelvis may be tilted and one leg longer than the other. Although many people suffering from scoliosis have found relief through yoga, if your curvature is very pronounced, consult your doctor or health specialist before beginning a yoga practice.

FOCUS ON: Lengthening the spine, working evenly on both sides.

POSES THAT MAY HELP: Ardha Chandrasana (Half-Moon Pose, Choudhury-style) and Trikonasana (Triangle Pose) with both feet turned forward; modified Downward-Facing Dog at the wall, lifting one leg at a time without disturbing the rest of the body; Basic Prone on hands and knees, lifting opposite arm to leg, while keeping the back flat.

Tips for Creating Good Posture and Proper Alignment

- Balance your weight from the floor up, and from foot to foot, or hip to hip.
- Adjust plumb line: earlobe, shoulder, hip, knee, and ankle.
- Focus inwardly: Be aware of the center of your body, around the navel area.
- Focus outwardly: Choose a point of focus on the floor or on the wall opposite you. Note that some poses will have a particular point of focus, *drishti,* on which to channel your attention.
- Cultivate sthira and sukha: Seek stability and comfort in the breath, postures, and movement.
- Use affirmations when you find your attention wandering: If you do Mountain Pose (Tadasana), for example, it may help to repeat silently, "I am strong, stretched, and centered. I am a mountain—tall, solid, and grand."

3

∞

Styles of Hatha Yoga—A Method For Every Body

You may have heard yoga classes referred to as "Iyengar," "Kundalini," "Kripalu," or "Sivananda" yoga. And you're probably wondering which one of these is hatha yoga. Actually, they all are. Each one is simply a *style* of hatha yoga. Many of these styles have specific characteristics which reflect a particular teacher's approach to asanas; others reflect the characteristics or teachings of a particular organization. For example, Iyengar is hatha yoga practiced in a manner prescribed by yoga master B. K. S. Iyengar; Kundalini yoga was developed by Yogi Bhajan, founder of 3HO; and Kripalu is the type of yoga Swami Amrit Desai brought to the United States in 1971. Some of these systems are quite vigorous, while others are less physically demanding and have a more meditative quality. Some emphasize breathing techniques along with asana, while still others focus on more individualized instruction or on yoga's therapeutic aspects.

One thing you may notice when you actually go out to experience some of these styles firsthand is that not only are the poses taught slightly differently from style to style, but the names may not even be the same. For instance, the Half-Moon Pose we've included from Choudhury's system differs radically from Iyengar's Half-Moon, which is an advanced one-legged balance that we have not included. Finally, you'll see that the English transliteration of Sanskrit terms will vary considerably from style to style.

While we don't pretend to offer a complete listing of all hatha yoga styles, the following will give you a sampling of the most widely practiced systems of hatha yoga today. Regardless of your age and fitness level, you'll no doubt find a style of yoga that will appeal to you and be most appropriate for your particular body or personality type. Later on in the book, you'll experience elements of many of these styles as we take you through a basic repertoire of breathing exercises and poses.

Iyengar Yoga/B. K. S. Iyengar

Probably the most widely recognized hatha yoga technique in the Western world, Iyengar-style yoga is both precise and dynamic. Iyengar teachers pay particularly close attention to the placement of the feet, hands, and pelvis, as well as to the alignment of the spine, arms, and legs. Because of this attention to detail, the pace of an Iyengar class tends to be slow to moderate.

The standing postures are emphasized, especially in beginning classes. Although you will undoubtedly be reminded to "breathe" in an Iyengar class, pranayama, or specific breathing techniques, are not taught in this method until the student attains a certain proficiency with the postures.

At one time dubbed the "furniture yogi" by his international students, Iyengar developed a number of yoga props—wood blocks and benches, sandbags, blankets, bolsters, and straps. Inspired by his teacher Krishnamacharya, Iyengar developed these aids as a support system to achieve greater symmetry and extension in the postures. For students who may be weak, very stiff, or have structural imbalances, this support system is extremely useful.

B. K. S. Iyengar, known as the "Lion of Pune" because of the strict nature of his technique and his own dynamic personality, is the author of *Light on Yoga,* as well as many other respected treatises in the field. He is also recognized for his profound knowledge and development of the therapeutic applications of hatha yoga. His school, the Ramamani Iyengar Memorial Yoga Institute, is dedicated to his late wife. Founded in 1974, and located in Pune, India, the institute attracts students from all over the world. His daughter Gita and son Prashant also teach yoga and help run and maintain his school.

There are numerous Iyengar yoga associations in America, as well as in Europe. These organizations support the continuance of the Iyengar method by sponsoring teachers for workshops and trainings. There are strict requirements for becoming a certified Iyengar yoga instructor.

Ashtanga Yoga/K. Pattabhi Jois

The Ashtanga *vinyasa* yoga system of K. Pattabhi Jois—not to be confused with the eightfold path or ashtanga yoga of Patañjali—is a rigorous practice, the intensity of which is comparable to the training of an elite athlete. In this system, vinyasa denotes a set sequence of poses. Characterized by a continual theme, or chorus, of jumping Sun Salutations that are performed between a variety of asanas, this is the most physically demanding of all the hatha yoga styles. The purpose of this continual flow of action is to create heat—or *tapas*—"to burn." This heating produces the cleansing or detoxifying effect associated with this method.

There are six sequences in total; the first series focuses on forward bends, with back-bending postures highlighting the second series. The other four series are very advanced; only an exceptionally small percentage of Jois's students have mastered these.

Ashtanga places equal emphasis on strength, flexibility, and stamina. Many fitness enthusiasts who thrive on intense workouts like this style. You will often find a higher ratio of men to women in an Ashtanga class.

Much to the dismay of the traditionalists of this form, you will sometimes see this system referred to as "power yoga." Ashtanga yoga classes, incarnated as power yoga and taught in modified fashion, have steadily increased in popularity in the past few years.

Jois's Ashtanga Yoga Institute is located in Mysore, India, where a steady stream of Americans and Europeans come to study. Jois has certified very few Westerners to teach Ashtanga yoga. Among them are Tim Miller, who directs The Ashtanga Yoga Center in Encinitas, California, and Richard Freeman, of Boulder, Colorado, who produced the video *Yoga with Richard Freeman: Ashtanga Yoga, The Primary Series*. Beryl Bender Birch, an Ashtanga/power yoga teacher based in New York City, has written a popular book entitled *Power Yoga*.

Viniyoga/T. K. V. Desikachar

This style is also referred to as yoga in the tradition of T. K. V. Desikachar, son of the late yoga master Krishnamacharya, and Iyengar's nephew. Based on the principle of *vinyasa krama*—which literally means an intelligently conceived, step-by-step approach to the teaching of asana—Viniyoga modifies and tailors the postures to the needs of the individual student.

The method of Viniyoga represents a kind of middle path between the precision of Iyengar yoga and the vigor of Ashtanga yoga. Distinguishing characteristics of this style include emphasis on the breath, a more relaxed approach to placement, a slower pace of execution, and a conscious application of yoga theory to asana practice. What this means is that in Viniyoga the importance of the breath takes precedence over form and execution of the poses. Breath and movement are consciously coordinated, and the inhalations and exhalations are articulated in varying lengths and ratios. Viniyoga teachers often set the pace with a metronome.

A more relaxed approach to placement means that the joints, especially the knees and elbows, are kept slightly bent. This allows the emphasis to be placed on extending the spine.

This system is often taught privately. Experienced Viniyoga instructors are likely to be well-versed in the therapeutic application of posture and breath, and they encourage open dialogue with their students, often focusing on yoga theory. Desikachar is based in Madras, India, where he heads the school named after his father, Krishnamacharya Yoga Mandiram.

Kundalini Yoga/Yogi Bhajan

In 1969 Yogi Bhajan, a Sikh from India, introduced Kundalini yoga to the West. This ancient practice is designed to awaken the Kundalini, or coiled energy, stored at the base of the spine. Through the use of breath, posture, chanting, and meditation, this energy is stimulated and consciously directed through the *chakras,* or energy centers, along the spine. Teachers of this method emphasize several breathing techniques. Among them are *nadhi shodhana* (literally, channel or nerve cleansing, accomplished through alternate nostril breathing), slow diaphragmatic breathing, and *agni pranayam* (breath of fire, also known as *kapalabhati*). Employing a dynamic approach to *kriyas* (cleansing and energizing techniques), Kundalini yogis combine various postures with the breath of fire.

Yogi Bhajan's Healthy, Happy, Holy Organization (3HO) is headquartered in Los Angeles and New Mexico. Focusing on the areas of health and healing, yogic lifestyle, vegetarian diet, and education, as well as community service, 3HO stresses family values in the truest sense of the word. It is designed for house-holders who lead active lives.

In 1996 there were nearly fifteen hundred Kundalini yoga teachers worldwide, primarily in the United States, Canada, Europe, Mexico, and South America. 3HO sponsors teacher training programs and yoga camps internationally and publishes *The Science of Keeping Up!* newsletter.

Kripalu Yoga/Yogi Amrit Desai

Developed by Yogi Amrit Desai, Kripalu yoga is characterized by its internally directed approach to asana practice. Desai's initial inspiration came from Kripalvananda, an Indian master of Kundalini yoga whose primary practice was actually pranayama.

Kripalu yoga has three stages. Within each stage, a student may experience a full range of intensity: gentle, moderate, and vigorous.

Stage 1, a willful practice to get you in touch with your body, teaches the basic mechanics of the postures including placement, alignment, and coordination of breath and movement. Teachers will encourage you to dis-cover your own strengths and weaknesses; where you hold tension, and the degree of your flexibility. Postures are held for relatively short durations—10–20 seconds.

Stage 2, referred to as will and surrender, introduces prolonged holding of the poses. It is at this stage that teachers will emphasize the monitoring of mental and emotional states. The meditative aspect is cultivated as you practice concentration and detachment.

Stage 3 becomes a surrendering to the wisdom of the body. This stage par-ticularly reflects Yogi Desai's own personal experience of performing the postures spontaneously, while being directed from his own internal aware-ness of Prana or life force energy. Desai called it a Meditation in Motion. At this stage, the practice becomes more interpretive, as teachers encour-age students to create the flow of their own practice. Within this third stage, a "go with the flow," non-competitive atmosphere presides, and goal setting is actively discouraged.

The Kripalu Center for Yoga and Health offers teacher training/certification programs at its center in Lenox, Massachusetts, as well as workshops, conferences, and retreats year-round.

Ananda Yoga/Swami Kriyananda

Ananda Yoga, developed by American J. Donald Walters and based at the Ananda community in Nevada City, California, is linked to Paramahansa Yogananda, author of *Autobiography of a Yogi*. Walters, also known as Swami Kriyananda, himself a disciple of Yogananda and a former Self Realization Fellowship (SRF) vice president, often publicly demonstrated Yogananda's approach to hatha yoga. That approach reflected Yogananda's kriya yoga techniques, the purpose of which was to clear and energize the system in preparation for meditation.

Walters left SRF in 1962 and founded the Ananda World Brotherhood Village, a residential community, in 1968. There he developed Ananda yoga. In this technique, each posture is viewed as a way to expand, or heighten, self-awareness. This process is enhanced through the use of affirmations, a distinctive feature of this system. For instance, the affirmation for Cobra is "I rise joyfully to meet each new opportunity." Another characteristic of this technique is the emphasis it places on deeply relaxing into the poses, keeping in mind that hatha is a preparation for meditation. Ananda also offers yoga teachers' training certification programs.

Yoga College of India–Choudhury Yoga/Bikram Choudhury

Known as the "yogi to the stars," Bikram Choudhury created a technique inspired by his teacher Bishnu Ghosh, the brother of Paramahansa Yogananda. An exact set of twenty-six postures with two pranayama techniques (one done at the beginning and the other at the end), this "beginners' class" is not so easy! Nearly all the postures are repeated twice and each is held for at least 10 seconds. An excellent routine for those already fit, considerations for injuries or sensitive backs are nominal.

Beginning with *ujjayi*—"the victorious breath"—the first part of the routine consists of standing postures and includes several challenging one-leg balances. The second part is done on the floor with backbends, forward bends, and twists making up this part of the session. *Kapalabhati*—"the breath of fire"—completes this series, followed by a brief relaxation. The thermostat will be set high—at least 80° or higher—and a humidifier is used as well.

For those who want even more challenge, Bikram offers an advanced workout; attendance in this class, however, is by invitation only.

Bikram's school, called Yoga College of India, first opened in Bombay in 1965. He has many locations including Tokyo, Honolulu, San Francisco, and Beverly Hills. Yoga teacher training certification programs are regularly conducted at the Beverly Hills location, where Bikram himself has been based since 1973.

Integral Yoga/Swami Satchidananda

Developed by Swami Satchidananda, the practice of Integral yoga reflects the teachings of his guru, Swami Sivananda (1887–1963), who taught a synthesis of many different types of yoga. As the name implies, Satchidananda's system is an integrative method incorporating yoga principles into lifestyle and thought. Devotees of this system are advised to be "easeful, peaceful, and useful." Ease in body, peace of mind, and usefulness in life are the guiding principles of Integral yoga.

Integral hatha yoga classes follow a set pattern and are 75 minutes in length. This format includes 45 minutes of asana, a deep relaxation, a pranayama sequence, and ends with a meditation. Although challenging, the feeling of the class is gentle and meditative and reflects a traditional approach that benefits all aspects of the individual.

An Indian by birth, Swami Satchidananda came to the United States at the behest of artist Peter Max in 1966. Delivering the opening talk at the Woodstock rock festival in 1969, Satchidananda became an inspiration to a whole generation of baby boomers, many of whom chanted their first "om" with him. He established the Integral Yoga Institute in 1966 (now called Integral Yoga International), which currently has over forty branches worldwide. The institute's headquarters is at Satchidananda Ashram–Yogaville in Buckingham, Virginia, a residential community of nearly one thousand acres.

Sivananda Yoga/Swami Vishnu-devananda

Another disciple of Swami Sivananda's and promoter of traditional hatha yoga was the late Swami Vishnu-devananda (1927–1993). After embarking on a 10-year intensive study of all aspects of yoga, Vishnu-devananda made his way to the West in 1958. Following brief stays in San Francisco, Miami, and New York City, he established the Sivananda Yoga Vedanta Centers in Montreal, Canada, in 1959. The Sivananda organization blossomed into an international entity with the success of Vishnu-devananda's *The Complete Illustrated Book of Yoga,* published in 1960, and his brilliant and innovative promotional skills.

Vishnu-devananda's system of yoga incorporates Sivananda's five-point method of practice, which includes proper exercise, breathing, deep relaxation, vegetarian diet, positive thinking, and meditation. Following a standard format, Sivananda's hatha yoga classes are based on a routine of breathing exercises, sun salutations, a series of twelve classic yoga postures, and relaxation. A short mantra chant and prayers begin and end each class.

In 1962, Vishnu-devananda founded the Sivananda Ashram Yoga Camp in Val Morin, Quebec, the first of six ashrams located in North America and India. The Sivananda Yoga Retreat, located in Nassau, Bahamas, is a favorite yoga getaway for yoga vacations as well as for Vishnu-devananda's four-week yoga teacher training course.

How to Find a Yoga Teacher (and Style) That's Right for You

The following guidelines will help you choose a teacher and the type of yoga that feels most comfortable for you.

- Consider your own needs and limitations as you go through the selection process.
- Consider your present physical condition and think about what you want to get out of the class.
- Ask the teacher about his or her training and credentials. Teacher training varies widely in depth and scope.

- Let the teacher know what you're looking for and get her advice on which classes you should take.
- Take classes in different styles until you find one that appeals to you.
- After taking a class, note your response: Did you have a rapport with the teacher? How did you feel before and after class? Was the intensity of the class about right?
- Appropriate responses to a class should be invigoration, calm, and satisfaction.
- Inappropriate responses would be stress, agitation, or physical discomfort.
- Once you find a method that works for you, stick with it!

PART 2

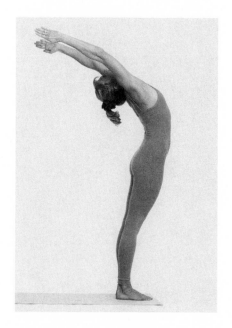

The Practice of Yoga

4

Breath: The Key to Health and Well-Being

According to modern science, we derive our energy from the food we eat and the water we drink, as well as from the air we take in as oxygen and dispel as carbon dioxide. All these ingredients provide the fuel we need to keep our bodies functioning. Key among them, of course, is oxygen. We can do without food and water for varying degrees of time, but obviously we cannot survive without air. In this Western view, energy is finite and measurable, something we need to constantly replenish. Hence, in this context, the breath serves a purely functional purpose: The air we inhale and exhale during respiration keeps us alive.

In Eastern thought, energy is a much broader concept, more than the food we eat and the air we breathe. While it is the very essence of those substances, it's not limited to them. Energy, or Prana as the yogis call it, and Chi as the Chinese refer to it, is everywhere and in limitless supply—all we have to do is open ourselves up as vehicles or channels for this omnipotent and omnipresent force. Words for energy or breath in this Eastern view include Prana, respiration, vitality, life, wind, strength, spirit, and soul. A proper flow and balance of this energy, which is carried by the breath, determines the state of our physical and spiritual health.

It's interesting to look at the origin of our words for the breath and notice the deeper meaning within them. The root word for respire is the Latin *spirare,* which means to breathe, but a derivative of *spirare, spiritus,* means the breath of a god. Other words that share the same root include inspire, aspire, and expire; examining their meanings we see a fuller understanding of the breath. To inspire, for example, means not only to take in air, but to stimulate the mind and emotions to produce specific feelings and actions. The definition of aspire (*ad* means more, above, or toward) is literally to breathe more or toward, but it is used to mean to strongly desire to be or do something lofty or grand. Expire, of course, means to bring to an end, to die. Its literal translation from the Latin is to run out of breath.

Spiritual Physiology

Yogis consider the body as a receptacle for Prana and our central nervous system the internal pathway for Prana. The central shaft of the spinal column is the main thoroughfare of this network. Called the *sushumna,* "most gracious" channel, it is the central conduit through which the pranic energy is directed. To the right of the spine is the *pingala,* "sun channel"; to the left is the *ida,* "moon channel." These three channels, called *nadis,* work together to direct the force of Prana throughout the body. The balance of the pingala and ida channels increases energy in the sushumna. In energetic terms, the balance of the nadis is the true essence, or source, of our health and vitality. Yogis believe that literally thousands of these channels exist in the body and that they connect to every tissue and every cell. Therefore, keeping the channels clear ensures the balanced flow of life force and results in optimal health.

A good way to understand the concept of Prana is to think of the body as a garden hose. If the hose is twisted or has kinks in it, the water cannot flow through it to nourish the garden. Similarly, when the body is misaligned or blocked by areas of tension or imbalance, Prana cannot flow freely. Another way of looking at Prana flow is to view the body as a system of electrical circuitry: The wires need to be kept clean, untangled, and properly connected in order for the current to flow and the lights and appliances to function properly.

Earlier in the book, we viewed Prana as having two complementary aspects: expansion, *brhmana,* and contraction, *langhana.* The yogis also define these aspects as *prana* (with a lower-case *p*) and *apana.* The first aspect, prana, stimulates the body to inhale. Although the inhalation appears to move down into the body, the action of prana is upward, light, energizing. It constitutes that part of the breath that fills up the body, moving along the right side, *pingala,* of the spine, creating heat and light, and invigorating the whole person. This prana, or solar energy, enters the body on the inhalation and during retention of the breath at the top of the inhalation. Its home in the body is in the torso, chest, and stomach area; it controls respiration and cardiovascular functioning. The energy you receive from this aspect is extroverted and active. The postures often associated with this expansion are backbends which hyperextend the spine and open up the chest.

Apana, or the lunar aspect of the vital energy, encourages the body to exhale. Although this aspect appears to be moving up and out of the body, because you're exhaling air, its action is downward, creating an anchoring effect. It moves down and through the body, along the left side, *ida,* of the spine, on the exhale or during suspension of the breath at the end of the exhalation. Centered in the lower torso, around the area of the colon and pelvis, apana controls digestion, assimilation processes, excretion, and sexual function. Apana energy is cold and dark, relaxing and pacifying, creating feelings of introspection and calm. As a result, apana-producing activities and poses are ideal for preparing for meditation. Postures often associated with introverted, or lunar energy, include the forward bends and twisting poses.

Mechanics of the Breath

The key muscles involved in respiration are the diaphragm; the intercostals, which are between the ribs; and the abdominal muscles encasing the front of the belly. Muscles in the neck, throat, chest, and upper back also engage, but less so.

The diaphragm, a huge double-dome-shaped muscle, is responsible for 75 percent of the respiratory process. Sitting in the chest like a parachute, the diaphragm attaches at the top to the sternum (the bottom of the breastbone); it travels down the sides of the body to the mid- to lower ribs, anchoring itself in the back to the first-to-fourth lumbar vertebrae of the lower spine. (Figure 6.) As we inhale, the diaphragm lowers and expands, and the breath draws in; when we exhale, this process is reversed. As we consciously engage both the abdominal and the intercostal muscles, supporting the movement of the diaphragm, the auxiliary muscles involved—in the chest, back, and neck—respond accordingly.

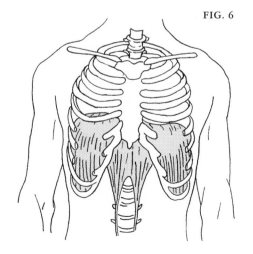

FIG. 6

Keep in mind that tension is the main culprit in blocking the flow of Prana and preventing us from breathing as properly or as fully as we could. The diaphragm is considered the seat of the emotions, and by learning deep diaphragmatic breathing, we learn to express our emotions more freely.

Using the Breath in Yoga Practice

Traditionally, a formal yoga practice would incorporate asanas before the pranayama practice. However, because we feel it's necessary to breathe properly in order to practice yoga asanas effectively, we've chosen to give you some breathing exercises before introducing you to the physical postures. This attention to the breath will further benefit you when you're feeling stressed or nervous, and when you begin your meditation practice.

Some styles of hatha yoga more actively incorporate pranayama techniques in their beginning classes than others. Viniyoga and Kundalini yoga both readily share pranayama exercises with their students from the start. B. K. S. Iyengar, on the other hand, believes a student must be thoroughly grounded in the asanas (completing four or five years of practice) before he or she adds pranayama to a daily routine.

Whether you learn pranayama or not in your yoga class, paying attention to your breathing will help to quiet your mind and deflect stress. As you come to be aware of your breathing, you'll find you can either stimulate your energy when it's low, or bring about a deep state of relaxation. Although you will learn specific breathing techniques in the next chapter, the following tips will help you in any yoga class you attend.

- Breathe abdominally. When you inhale, allow your belly to expand; when you exhale, consciously draw your navel in toward your spine by contracting your lower abdominals.
- Lengthen and equalize your breaths. As you breathe abdominally, you'll notice that your breaths get longer. Begin to consciously lengthen them, making the inhalation as long as the exhalation.
- Breathe in and out through the nose. At first you may find this difficult, especially if you have any kind of restriction in your nasal passages.

With regular practice you'll get better at it, and in time it'll become second nature to you.

- When in doubt, just breathe! Don't get overly concerned with how you're breathing. Remember, the breath is a tool we can use to enhance our practice and well-being, it's not an element to obsess over. After all, you're doing yoga to relieve stress, not create more!

Breath Retention and Suspension

After you get used to breathing from the belly, equalizing the breath, and breathing in and out through your nose, the next step is to pause consciously at the end of the inhalation. This is called breath retention and helps create the expansive qualities of heat and energy in the body. Then try pausing at the end of your exhalation—this is called breath suspension and activates the more pacifying qualities of coolness and relaxation. At the beginning, keep these pauses brief, no longer than five seconds each. To practice these for longer durations, seek the guidance of an experienced teacher.

Coordinating Breath and Movement

By learning to coordinate your breath with your movements, you'll find that you feel much more at ease in the poses. The rules governing whether you inhale or exhale—and when—are dictated by the direction in which the spine or limbs move. After you get the hang of it, the marriage of breath and movement will become second nature.

On the Inhalation: Inhalations are generally mated with upward or expanding movements. Going into a backbend such as Cobra, for example, you begin on an in-breath. Then you simply hold the pose and breathe rhythmically. An exception to this rule: Upward movements of the legs work best on the exhalation since the legs are much heavier than the arms.

On the Exhalation: Exhalations are usually mated with downward and contracting movements, such as lowering the arms, and with any positions that employ flexion of the spine (i.e., folding the body into itself such as in forward bends, abdominal curls, lateral stretches, or twists). When you lift a substantial weight, exhale on the effort. This applies whether you're lifting a 10-pound dumbbell or your leg. The out-breath helps contract the abdominals which in turn stabilize and protect the lower back.

Imagery and Visualization

Imagery can help encourage the flow or the direction of your breath. Regardless of what posture you're holding or what direction you're moving in, visualize lengthening your spine and opening your chest with each inhalation. Feel that you are moving up and out, literally expanding. With each exhalation, take the opportunity to re-anchor and draw your energy down and inward. This will help you reconnect to your center—the pelvic region—and strengthen the abdominals.

Breath Awareness Techniques

Based on the principles of yoga, the following exercises reflect both the philosophical as well as the mechanical aspects of the breath. This series also includes exercises on coordinating breath and movement and will effectively equip you with a variety of simple techniques you can access at any time. You will learn how to breathe in a manner that will promote relaxation and help you to manage stress. Additionally, we have included techniques which will boost your energy level.

In general, any one of these techniques or any combination of them may be considered a preparation for contemplative activity or actual meditation practice. These exercises are effective and safe for virtually everyone; however, if any of these exercises make you feel uncomfortable in any way, simply stop and return to normal breathing.

These exercises condition the muscles involved in the respiratory process. Just as it takes time to become stronger and more flexible in your poses, it takes time—and practice—to develop breath awareness. It is also important to keep in mind the intricate connection that the breath has to our emotions, the nervous system, and our psychological state of being. Whether intentional or not, stress placed upon our breathing patterns interferes with both our mental and physical well-being. So please, relax and enjoy all the following exercises.

On the Floor Breath Exercises

You'll do the first three exercises supine, which means lying on the floor on your back. Bend your knees and place your feet hip distance apart. Place a small folded towel under your head so that your neck is in an extended or neutral position in line with the rest of the spine. Arms will remain at your sides with your palms either facing up or down. We will refer to this placement as your "Basic Supine."

EXERCISE #1: Observance of the Breath

Close your eyes. (Figure 7.) Begin by observing your natural breathing process. Don't change it in any way; simply observe it. What moves in your body when you breathe? Your chest and/or shoulders? Your ribs and/or abdomen? Do you notice any particular area or areas of tension, perhaps in the neck or even the face, or maybe in the abdominal area and pelvis? Are you breathing through your mouth, your nose, or a combination of both? Is your breath short or long? What is the ratio—that is, the count or length of your inhalation in relation to the exhalation? Do you tend to hold your breath, either in or out? Allow yourself a couple of minutes for this process.

Now that you have a sense of your normal breathing pattern and how you "naturally" breathe, you can begin to extend the breath. During the following exercises, keep your eyes open, softly focus your gaze, and keep your facial muscles relaxed. In between exercises, close your eyes, relax, and breathe normally—a

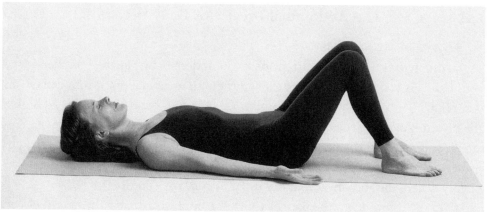

FIG. 7

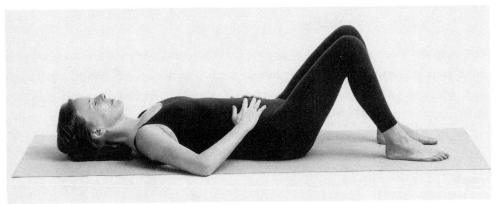

FIG. 8

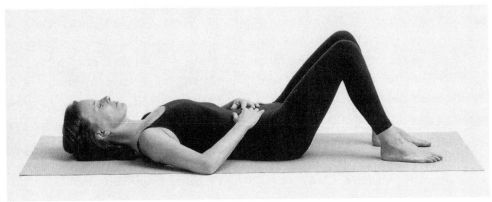

FIG. 9

good time to "tune in" and reflect upon your response to the previous exercise. Breathe in and out through the nose unless otherwise instructed.

EXERCISE #2: The Abdominal Breath (or Belly Breathing)

POSITION: Basic Supine.

TECHNIQUE: Bring your attention to the abdomen by placing your hands over your belly. As you inhale, begin to expand the abdomen, making it rounded or convex, allowing the breath to gently push it up into your hands. (Figure 8.) Think of the breath expanding into your lower back and into the sides of the abdomen. You are expanding in all directions from the center of your pelvis. As you breathe out, gently press the belly downward with your hands, allowing the exhalation to completely deflate the abdomen, making it flat or concave. (Figure 9.)

PACING: Slow down the pace of your breathing, equalizing the length of your inhalation and your exhalation. You may want to count a rhythm silently that is comfortable for you, such as 5 counts in, and 5 counts out.

EMPHASIS: Now shift your attention to the exhalation, first making it longer than your inhalation. It need only be a second or two longer. Next, emphasize the out-breath even more by pausing at the end of the exhalation. Again, this will be mild, simply suspending the breath for a few counts.

IMAGE: With each exhalation imagine that you are letting go of any tension you noticed while observing the breath in the previous exercise.

REPETITIONS: Practice each stage of this exercise for several breaths—anywhere from 3 to 7 repetitions.

RESULTS: Deep abdominal, diaphragmatic breathing has a calming effect on the entire system. It massages the organs of the abdominal area and enhances their functions. Although you needn't breathe like this all the time, or even expand the belly to this degree throughout your whole practice, this is the most important and useful of all these breath awareness techniques. It is also the first stage of abdominal strengthening. Each time you emphasize the exhalation you engage a substantial portion of the lower abdominal musculature.

EXERCISE #3: The Chest Breath (or Heart/Thoracic Breathing)

POSITION: Basic Supine.

TECHNIQUE: Return to deep abdominal breathing while shifting your awareness to the center of the chest. We will repeat the same process here that we established with Belly Breathing: lengthening the breath and creating equality in the timing of the inhalation and exhalation. (Figure 10.)

FIG. 10

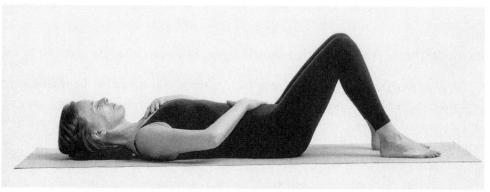

PACING: Again, establish a rhythm that is comfortable—3 to 5 counts in, and 3 to 5 counts out.

EMPHASIS: Emphasize the inhalation by breathing up into the center of the chest. Think of expanding to the front, sides, and back of the chest with each inhalation. Then lengthen the inhalation, making it slightly longer than the exhalation. When you are ready, hold the breath in for a few moments at the completion of your inhalation.

IMAGE: With each inhalation, imagine that you are drawing in the energy that nourishes you. Think positively, breathe in all thoughts and feelings that uplift and empower you such as joy, health, and abundance.

REPETITIONS: 3 to 7 repetitions for each stage of this exercise.

RESULTS: This technique will be more stimulating than Belly Breathing. Although you are still breathing abdominally, the additional emphasis placed on the chest and the inhalation is energizing.

You have now experienced the first stages of breath awareness. You have a sense of the muscular activity involved in the respiratory process, and you have begun to consciously participate in extending or directing your breath. The next three techniques are part of the classical pranayama repertoire. The first technique—*ujjayi,* or victorious breath—introduces the element of sound to the breath. The second technique—*kapalabhati,* or "breath of fire"—both energizes and cleanses. Finally, we have included a yoga *mudra,* a technique which emphasizes the exhalation and has a calming, sedative effect on the system. You may practice all three of these seated in a chair, or if you like, try them on the floor "yoga style." (For instructions on the basic seated floor posture, *Sukhasana,* refer to the chapter on asana.) Again, keep the eyes open with a soft gaze directed to the floor. You may close them when you rest and breathe normally in between the exercises.

EXERCISE #4: Breath with Sound–*Ujjayi*–Victorious Breath

DESCRIPTION: The prefix *ud* attached to verbs and nouns in Sanskrit means upward or superiority in rank. It denotes blowing or expanding and suggests pre-eminence and power. *Jaya* means conquest, victory, triumph, or success and implies restraint or curbing. As you breathe in and out through the nose, you create a sound by drawing the breath to the back of the throat which you have narrowed by contracting the epiglottis. One of the most fundamental of all yogic breathing modalities, ujjayi is practiced on its own and incorporated into virtually all of the pranayama repertoire. Some styles of hatha yoga encourage its use during asana practice, while others pay little attention to it, relegating this technique exclusively to pranayama.

POSITION: Seated in a chair, or on the floor.

TECHNIQUE: Allow your breathing to come into its own comfortable rhythm, breathing in and out through the nose. Imagine the back of the throat as a straw. Sip the breath into this straw as though you were drinking the air with your throat. You should feel the incoming air on the soft palate at the back of the throat and hear it as it makes a sibilant sound (sa). Similarly, on the exhale, you'll feel the breath at the back of the throat and hear it make an aspirate sound (ha).

PACING: Moderate to slow—3 to 5 counts in, 3 to 5 counts out.

EMPHASIS: On physical balance and mental equanimity. Listening to this sound is one of the ways we can "read" the body: A smooth, even sound indicates calm; a rough, uneven sound suggests agitation or imbalance.

IMAGE: The sound that the breath creates is not unlike the sound of the ocean at a distance. Many teachers suggest imitating the breath of "Darth Vader," the *Star Wars* character. Although this is far louder than your ujjayi breath needs to be, this exaggeration may help you to accomplish this technique more easily.

REPETITIONS: Practice one to two minutes at a time. Ultimately, you'll be able to sustain ujjayi breathing throughout your yoga practice.

RESULTS: Ujjayi draws more oxygen into the lungs and increases endurance. It reduces phlegm and strengthens the immune system. As the name "victorious breath" implies, this technique is empowering, enhancing the respiratory system and soothing—or gaining "victory"—over the nervous system.

NOTE: The final two techniques introduce a greater degree of breath control. Wait until you feel comfortable and proficient with the previous techniques before adding these to your repertoire. Do not attempt them at all if you are pregnant, have high or low blood pressure, or suffer from ear congestion or eye complaints (detached retina or glaucoma).

EXERCISE #5: Breath of Fire–*Kapalabhati*–Skull Lustre

DESCRIPTION: *Kapala* means skull. *Bhati* is translated as light or lustre. In this "skull brightening" technique the exhalation is forceful and active while the inhalation is passive. Often referred to as the "breath of fire," this cleansing breath

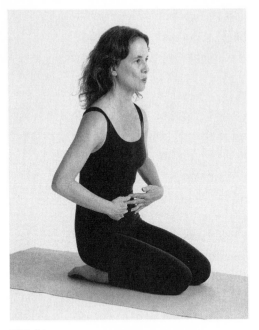

FIG. 11

is heat producing and stimulating. Initially, exhale through your mouth, as Bikram Choudhury teaches it. This helps you coordinate the contraction of your abdominal muscles with your exhalations. After you get the hang of it, exhale through the nose instead, which is the traditional technique.

POSITION: Kneel on the floor in what is called *vajrasana,* the "thunderbolt pose," or sit in a chair. Place your hands palms down on your thighs. Your back should be straight with the shoulders rolled back and down. Keep the abdominal area totally unrestricted.

TECHNIQUE: Take a deep breath in. Round your lips and begin to blow the breath out through your mouth by strongly contracting your abdominal musculature. (Figure 11.) As you release your abdomen, the breath will be drawn in again. Each exhalation should be directed and powerful; your inhalations will take care of themselves.

PACING: Each exhalation should be about one second ("one, one thousand") in duration. As you become more experienced you may quicken your pace.

EMPHASIS: On the exhalation and on the strong abdominal contractions of the lower belly. Keep your eyes absolutely focused on one spot during the entire exercise. The rest of the body remains passive.

IMAGE: Imagine that you are blowing out candles on a birthday cake placed several feet in front of you.

REPETITIONS: Repeat 20 to 40 times, ultimately building up to 60 repetitions per set and practicing for two sets. Rest in between your sets and breathe normally.

RESULTS: In addition to the benefits to the respiratory system, this exercise massages the abdominal organs, strengthens the abdominal wall, and tapers the waistline. It has a stimulating effect on the entire system.

CAUTION: If you feel a little light-headed or dizzy, simply stop and return to normal breathing. This dizziness happens because of the increase of oxygen that this exercise produces. Ultimately your system will adjust.

EXERCISE #6: **Yoga *Mudra*–Seal of Union**

DESCRIPTION: *Yoga* means union and *mudra* is a seal or hand gesture. This breathing technique is practiced with movement from a seated posture with the emphasis placed on the exhalation. It has a quieting effect on the mind and gently tones the abdomen. This modified version is one of many yoga mudras in the hatha yoga repertoire.

POSITION: Sit in Sukhasana or upright at the edge of a chair. Arms are behind your back. Hold either wrist with the opposite hand. (Figure 12.)

TECHNIQUE: Begin upright. Empty the lungs by blowing the breath out through the mouth. From here onward, breathe through your nose. Incorporate the ujjayi breath, only if you feel comfortable doing so. Keep the spine straight and inhale. Incline forward as you exhale, moving from the hips (not the waist). (Figure 13.) You need only come forward about 30 to 45 degrees. It is more important that the spine remains straight than that you come all the way forward. Hold at this angle, suspending the breath. That is, after you have emptied the lungs and inclined forward, hold the position without breathing for several seconds.

FIG. 12

FIG. 13

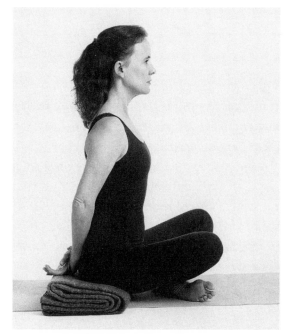

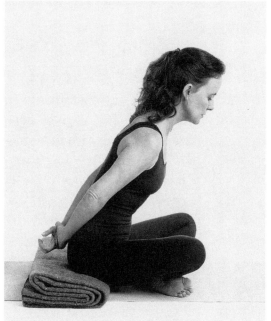

Draw your abdominal area in and up—from the pubic bone to the navel. As you return upright, inhale. Remain in your neutral or beginning position as you exhale. You have completed one round of this variation of yoga mudra. If you feel that you need to, breathe a few normal breaths before you repeat this exercise. Note that one round consists of two full breaths, holding the breath out after the first exhalation.

PACING: The pace should be moderate, one that you can manage without feeling that you have to gasp for breath in between rounds. The exhalation should be slightly longer than the inhalation. For instance, if you inhale for 3 or 4 counts, then exhale for 5 or 6 counts. The breath is then held out at the end of the exhalation for as long as you are comfortable, no longer than 5 counts.

EMPHASIS: On the exhalation and maintaining a straight spine.

IMAGE: Imagine that each exhalation lets go of all negative thoughts and feelings.

REPETITIONS: Practice for 3 to 5 repetitions. As your stamina improves you can perform your repetitions in succession, without resting in between efforts. Other ways to make this exercise more challenging are to either lengthen the count without adding repetitions, or keep the same count and add repetitions.

RESULTS: Yoga mudra calms the nervous system, strengthens the back, and tones the abdominal organs.

Standing Breath Exercises

We have already indicated the importance of keeping the spine supple by taking it through its full range of motion on a regular basis and explained how to coordinate the breath with movement. The following exercises combine these principles in a series of standing stretches. In addition to demonstrating the mechanics of breath and movement, this sequence is an excellent warm-up before a practice (especially of standing poses) and works well as a mini routine that you can do any time. It is an especially useful sequence following long periods of sitting at a desk or in a car. Consider it an essential part of your repertoire. Practice all these movements in "Basic Stance"—that is, standing with feet hip-distance apart, knees slightly bent, and arms at your sides.

EXERCISE #7: **Standing Cobra**

DESCRIPTION: This exercise demonstrates the principle of inhaling and hyperextending or arching the spine.

POSITION: Basic Stance.

TECHNIQUE: On an inhale, stretch your arms behind you, clasping your hands. Interlace the fingers with the palms facing one another. Pause here and exhale. Keep your buttocks firm, your tail tucked under, and your knees soft. Continue to breathe rhythmically. Straighten your elbows and, keeping your hands clasped, draw your arms away from your buttocks. Inhale and lift the chest, raising your chin slightly. Gently arch backward and look up. Pause here and exhale. Hold here for a few breaths. On an inhale lift into the chest; keep this lift as you exhale, press into your hands, and continue to tuck the tailbone under. (Figure 14.) When you are ready, bring your upper torso back to center, release your hands, and allow your arms to return to your sides.

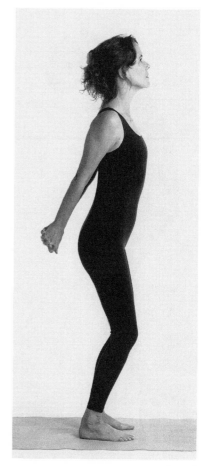

FIG. 14

PACING: Move into this movement slowly and take several breaths to complete this exercise.

EMPHASIS: On the inhalation and on breathing into the chest. Focus on the stretch through the chest, rib cage, and into the arms.

IMAGE: Imagine Cobra Pose done upright (see asana section). As you increase the distance from the pubic bone to the navel and from the navel to the sternum, the back muscles contract and shorten. However, you are not compressing the lower back. Rather, you are lifting out of the lower back by continually lifting the chest upward while tucking the tailbone down and under.

REPETITIONS: Doing this once or twice as a warm-up is sufficient. It is also a good movement to do anytime during a standing routine as a stabilizing exercise.

RESULTS: This exercise enhances respiration and is stimulating. It tones the arms and back, improves posture, and stretches the muscles of the chest. As in all back-bending poses, we are opening up both physically and emotionally when we practice this stretch.

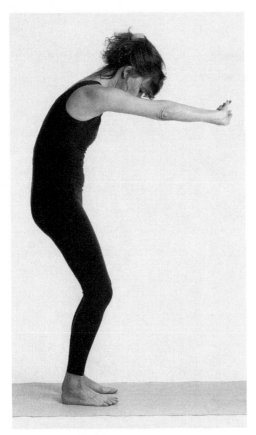

FIG. 15

EXERCISE #8: Standing Cat

DESCRIPTION: Here we emphasize the exhalation as we experience forward flexion. You will contract the front of the body as you lengthen the back of the body.

POSITION: Basic Stance.

TECHNIQUE: Bring your arms forward with elbows straight and clasp your hands in front of you at chest level, palms facing toward you and knuckles facing away from you. Inhale. As you exhale, simultaneously bend your knees, turn your palms away from you, and round your spine. Your arms remain parallel to the floor. Look down at your chest. (Figure 15.) Hold here and breathe for several breaths.

PACING: Move slowly into this stretch and hold it for several breaths.

EMPHASIS: On the exhalation. As you inhale think of separating your shoulder blades; when you exhale draw your navel up toward your backbone. Focus on the length you are creating in your back while you flatten the abdomen and decrease the distance from the pubic bone to the sternum.

IMAGE: Imagine closing into yourself. Cultivate the feeling of drawing into your center—the navel area.

REPETITIONS: Do this once or twice as a prep, anytime as an isolated stretch, or as a stabilizing stretch during a standing routine of poses.

RESULTS: Relieves tension in the upper back. Tones the abdominal area internally and externally.

EXERCISE #9: Modified Half-Moon

DESCRIPTION: This is a modified version of, and preparation for, a posture you will do later in the chapter on asana. The spine will be stretched to the side or laterally flexed in this two-part exercise.

POSITION: Basic Stance.

TECHNIQUE:

Stage 1: Inhale and interlace your fingers in front of you at chest level, palms facing toward you. As you exhale, turn your palms away and bring your arms above your head. Your palms are now facing up toward the ceiling. Keep your knees bent, buttocks firm, and the tail tucked under. As you straighten your elbows, drop your shoulders away from your earlobes, and soften the throat. Keep your arms in line with your head. If you feel tightness in your neck, shoulders, or lower back, bend your elbows. (Figure 16.) Hold here for 2 or 3 breaths. As you

FIG. 16

FIG. 17

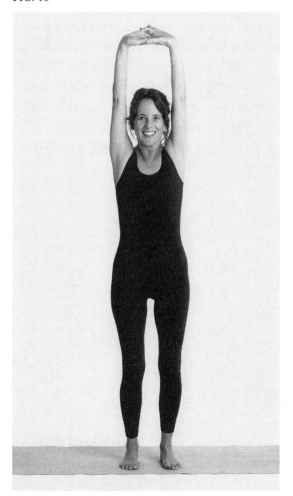

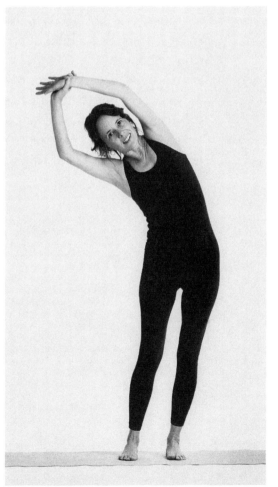

inhale, press upward into your hands. Lengthen your torso, separating your lower ribs from the tops of your hips. As you exhale, draw your navel toward your backbone. Extend through the backs of your legs down toward your heels.

Stage 2: Unclasp your hands and take hold of your left wrist with your right hand. Inhale and straighten your left elbow, keeping the right elbow slightly bent. As you exhale bend directly to the right. Keep your knees bent and tailbone tucked under. (Figure 17.) Hold here for a few breaths. Inhale as you lift upright. Exhale. Inhale and hold your right wrist with your left hand and reverse the stretch. To complete, come upright on the inhalation. Exhale as you release your arms down to your sides. Pause in place for a few breaths.

PACING: Move slowly into this stretch and hold each stage for two to three breaths.

EMPHASIS: In Stage 1, focus on lengthening the torso, including the arms. In Stage 2, focus on bending directly to the side, engaging the abdominals as you return to center.

IMAGE: Lengthening out of the crown of your head and thinning the waist.

REPETITIONS: Once or twice as a prep; anytime as an isolated stretch, or as a stabilizing exercise during your daily routine.

RESULTS: This pose prepares you for all lateral (side-bending) postures. It tones the abdominals and tapers the waist.

5

Guidelines for Practice

There is very little you need to do in order to practice yoga. Think of it more as being ready and present. Yoga is essentially a process in which you continually allow yourself to unfold, rather than strive to achieve a particular goal or level of accomplishment. If there is any goal at all in this process, it would be to allow yourself the experience of "being" rather than of doing or having.

Contrary to popular belief, you need not be flexible in order to begin your study of yoga, although you will certainly become more flexible with consistent practice. It is also not mandatory to sit in Lotus or to stand on your head! Although very beneficial, these postures are for more advanced students.

You need not adhere to strict dietary demands; you don't even have to become a vegetarian. With continued study, however, you may find that your tastes and appetites change and fresh, natural, wholesome foods become more appealing to you. Some students have enjoyed a reduction in caloric and fat intake without even consciously trying!

All you really need in order to begin your practice is to be open, empty, and bare—that is, come with an open mind, an empty stomach, and bare feet.

Open Mind

An ancient story illustrates the open mind concept beautifully. A student comes to a teacher, requesting to be trained. As they talk, the student tries to impress the master with the knowledge he has already acquired, telling him how he wishes to be taught and what he needs to learn. As he listens, the teacher begins to pour tea into the student's cup. He continues pouring, seemingly oblivious to the fact that the cup is full. Soon the cup overflows, spilling the tea all over the floor. Finally, the exasperated student protests, "Sir, can you not see that the cup is full?" To which the master replies, "Ah, but is this cup not just like you—already filled to the brim? I cannot teach someone whose cup is already full. You must empty yourself so that you may receive some small amount of what I have to offer you." You too must approach your practice with a beginner's mind—one that is open and ready to receive.

Empty Stomach

As with any exercise, it is best to practice yoga on an empty stomach. Wait at least two to three hours after a large meal, and one to two hours after a lighter one before beginning. If you feel you need some "fuel" before a session, or if you have a tendency to get low blood sugar, have a little fruit, yogurt, or a protein drink up to an hour before practice. Note that internal pressure on the organs increases with the practice of asanas, so having a full stomach, bladder, or bowels could prove quite uncomfortable and even cause you to feel dizzy or nauseous.

Bare Feet

Bare feet are ideal when you practice yoga and actually serve a dual purpose. First and foremost, you need to have traction for the standing poses so that you won't slip. Secondly, working without shoes helps you fully exercise and articulate your feet. Let your feet breathe! An exception to this rule would be if you are doing a practice exclusively on the floor (supine or prone) and you need socks for warmth. Of course, if you must wear orthotics in your athletic shoes, or if you are practicing yoga outside after an aerobic activity, then by all means, keep your shoes on.

Observe, Accept, Be Patient

Yoga constantly encourages us to expand our awareness. Expanding our awareness involves developing the ability to see or observe with clarity; in yoga this is called *svadhyaya,* or self-study.

Before we can bring about changes for the better, or improve any condition, we must be aware of what's happening at the moment. With this awareness comes a sense of detachment. In other words, we don't judge our condition, or even our progress, we just notice it. For instance, you may realize that your right hip is a great deal tighter than your left. That's neither bad nor good—it just is. Learning to accept what is will better equip you to take action to rebalance and realign, to bring harmony where there may have been disharmony.

With acceptance actually comes a kind of empowerment. Recognizing your special uniqueness, your individuality, gives you an opportunity to change the frustration or dissatisfaction you feel into acceptance of who you are and where you are right now. Cultivating this attitude can energize and propel you on your path. With this acceptance comes the third component in this equation: patience.

Just as we view a baby with love, accepting that she will fall and get up many times as she learns how to walk, we can look at ourselves in this same way. Being patient with yourself will not only take the pressure off having to get to a certain goal within a certain length of time—allowing you to really enjoy your practice—but it's a great way to prevent injuries.

Being Safe: Considerations and Contraindications

Following the guidelines on attitude and acceptance we just recommended, as well as the logistics of practice, creates a framework of mindfulness within your daily yoga routine. To ensure that your practice feels safe and appropriate, especially when you're first beginning, we'd like to offer a few more tips.

Listening to Your Body

Because yoga can be such an effective tool for self-transformation, there is the temptation to get impatient and overuse its power. Remember, let moderation be the key and common sense your motto.

We develop the abilities to be moderate and use our common sense best by listening to our bodies, or developing what we call an "internal dialogue." Our bodies constantly give us signals to attend to. When we feel acute pain or extreme fatigue our body is telling us—in no uncertain terms—that we need to heed its signals. These cues are obvious ones and easy to focus on. But in yoga we also learn to listen to a quieter, more subtle communication that goes on all the time. Listening to our breathing, taking note of our energy level, acknowledging our emotional state each time we approach our practice will help us create the harmony we seek through yoga. Essentially what this all means is: If it's painful, **stop!** Discontinue the move or pose causing you pain. If you feel exhausted, **rest!** Back off a bit; perhaps skip yoga entirely for the day, or treat your body to a more restorative practice involving breathing, relaxation, and meditation techniques instead.

Discernment

Knowing how to distinguish pain from intensity and fatigue from lethargy is difficult at first, but paying attention to the breath can help. If your breath begins to feel unsteady, you're probably going beyond your present limits, are feeling some pain or acute discomfort, and are increasing your chances for injury. When your breath is steady, you still feel the intensity of the posture but without creating any pain or injury. Similarly, if you're overly tired or not feeling well, your breath will reflect that, becoming shallow and erratic. But if you're simply low in energy or a bit lethargic because you're lacking in oxygen, slow, deep breathing can enliven you, and you'll end your practice feeling much better than when you began.

Contraindications

Certain postures and breathing techniques may be recommended to remedy specific structural conditions and physiological functions. Conversely, there are poses and breathing techniques which should not be done in certain circumstances. Here's a list of the most common conditions, along with the postures, movements, and breathing techniques to avoid when these conditions are present:

Condition	Sciatica
Do Not Do	Forward bends or intense stretching of hamstrings
Condition	Menstruation
Do Not Do	Inverted postures
Condition	Hypertension/high blood pressure
Do Not Do	Breath retentions or inverted poses

Condition	Glaucoma, other eye problems, or ear congestion
Do Not Do	Breath retentions or inverted poses
Condition	Pregnancy
Do Not Do	Breath retentions or suspensions, as they limit the flow of blood to the fetus; inversions

The Use of Props

When you first get started in your practice, using a folded blanket, a strap, a chair, a block, or even the wall offers great support—literally—in many of the postures. These items, which you can usually find around the house, can help accommodate the tightness and weaknesses that plague most adults in our Western culture. Because we sit so much of the time—at our desks and in our cars—and because our dress habits—wearing shoes and carrying items on one shoulder or hip—cause postural imbalances, the tightness and weaknesses that develop make even some of the most basic yoga postures extremely challenging. So, at least in the beginning, if you use props to modify the postures to accommodate your body, you'll be able to experience the symmetry and correct alignment of the pose sooner. Then, as you become stronger, more centered, and more flexible, you'll find yourself less dependent upon the props. The following are the props most commonly used in yoga classes and for home practice.

Blanket

A firmly woven blanket, folded and placed underneath the hips, works well for seated postures done on the floor and is particularly beneficial for those of us who experience tightness in the hips, lower back, and hamstrings.

Strap

An old bathrobe belt is ideal; thick elastic resistance bands used in fitness classes and by physical therapists work well too. Mainly, the use of the strap helps stretch the hamstrings in either a seated or supine position.

Chair

A standard metal folding chair or a straight-back wooden chair with no arms works best. Simply sitting at the front edge of the chair, with legs uncrossed and feet flat on the floor, builds strength in the back muscles. The chair is useful for seated breathing exercises and meditation, is highly recommended as an alternative to sitting on the floor, and provides support when you're learning standing poses. It offers an excellent option for people with sensitive knees since many of the poses can be modified to be done using a chair. If your feet don't rest flat on the floor comfortably when you're sitting on the chair, place a folded blanket, a couple of blocks, or even two books of equal height underneath them.

Blocks

Yoga teachers use wooden blocks for support in a variety of ways. If your hamstrings are tight, for example, and you can't rest your hands on the ground near your feet in Forward Bend, resting each one on a separate block allows you to experience the benefits of the stretch without hurting yourself. In lieu of wooden blocks, use a telephone directory or any thick book.

The Wall

Even the wall can be considered a prop or a means of support. Some students even see it as a kind of teacher that checks and corrects our alignment. No matter what part of the body is touching the wall, we can use its contact or reference point to create symmetry and balance in a whole variety of postures.

Other Props

Some yoga teachers—particularly from the Iyengar tradition—add several other types of props to their repertoire: eye bags, bolsters, and sandbags. Improvise with household substitutes or check out mail-order companies that sell ready-made yoga props. For students with extra sensitive knees, a folded towel underneath the knees—or even actual athletic knee pads—bring welcome relief.

Preparing for Practice

The asanas we have chosen for this book provide you with a basic repertoire on which to build your practice and study. An eclectic blend, these poses reflect many of the different styles of hatha yoga we have previously described. In addition they address the fundamental aspects of asana: range of motion of the spine, pose and counterpose, postures to increase energy and those conducive to relaxation.

Beginning on the floor, we will take you through a series of poses that will bring awareness to your spine, creating mobility and stabilization in the torso, while addressing range of motion in both the hip and shoulder joints. You will then progress through a series of standing postures and one-leg balances, emphasizing strength, flexibility, stamina, and balance.

Returning to the floor, you'll practice a number of seated postures which will again focus your attention on the strength of your back while addressing the flexibility in the hip joints and hamstrings. Within this framework, you'll become aware of torsion of the spine as well as abdominal strength and get a chance to experience inversions. Finally, we'll introduce you to the Sun Salutation which you can incorporate into your daily routine or use as a separate practice. Note that there is logic to this progression: Each posture prepares you for the next pose, each segment of this progression complements the previous one. We'll suggest modifications and options for each pose, and, where appropriate, offer levels or stages.

Before you get started, we've included some general guidelines to help you get the most benefit from your yoga practice.

- Seek that balanced state of sthira and sukha—stability and comfort—in all of the postures.
- Do not strain or force. As with any exercise routine, it's important to start slowly, accelerating your pace and adding more challenging poses when you feel ready.
- Keep your eyes open.
- Although we will be cuing you on the breath as you move into and out of the postures, in the interim, just breathe!

Positional Cues

Here are a few examples of common directions that you may encounter in any given yoga class as well as in our instructions to the postures:

Contract, or Engage. Involves a tightening of the musculature in any given posture or movement. Note that engaging a muscle is different than gripping it. You merely want to activate the muscle, not overtax it or cause undue fatigue.

Release, Soften. The opposite of engaging, this movement is the conscious relaxation of the muscle. Directing specific areas to soften or let go also helps to relieve chronic areas of tension or "knots." These are areas that we tend never to release, ones that maintain a constant "holding pattern" of tension. "Soften your knees and elbows" means to bend these joints slightly.

Stacking & Tracking. These both refer to maintaining balanced and congruent alignment of the spine and the joints. Stacking most often refers to static alignment—how your spine "stacks up" when you're still: earlobe, shoulder, hip, knee, and ankle, all aligned in the vertical or upright context. This is what is meant by "plumb line" or neutral spine. Tracking refers to keeping this alignment in agreement as your body moves through space. For example, when you bend your knees, they should remain in alignment with your hips and ankles.

Breathing Into. This refers to directing your attention to the area of the body that is being activated or emphasized in any given movement or posture. This "breathing into" keeps your attention focused on what you want to accomplish (i.e., breathing into the back of your legs when you are practicing a forward bend keeps you focused on the hamstrings, the muscles that we want to stretch in this particular posture).

Tucking Under. This is a common direction that refers to drawing the tailbone down and forward to lengthen the lower back. This is particularly useful to anchor the lower body in backbends. Conversely, in forward bends you would release the tailbone back, the opposite of tucking under. Don't overdo the tucking under—you merely want to anchor the pelvis with this action, not restrict your movements!

Sit Bones. The sit bones are the tuberosities of the *ischia,* the lowest points of your pelvis. When you sit properly, these points touch the floor.

Tweezing the Buttocks. This action draws the sit bones together, which engages the buttocks and the hamstrings.

Now let's practice!

6

Supine Poses

We'll begin our instruction with the supine postures which promote flexibility. These poses, together with the prone postures, will put you in touch with the range of motion in your pelvis, hips, and shoulder joints, as well as the articulation of your spine. The beginning position for these poses is what we call "Basic Supine," the same position you took for the supine breathing exercises in chapter 4. Lie on your back with your legs bent and feet hip-distance apart (approximately 6 to 8 inches). (Figure 18.) Place a small folded towel under your head so the neck and head are in line with the rest of the spine. Relax your facial muscles, drop your shoulders away from your earlobes, and keep the back of the neck long. You're ready to practice.

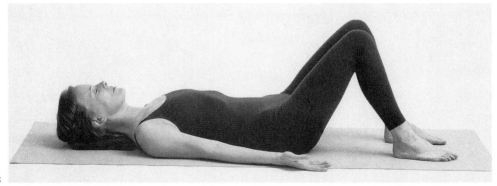

FIG. 18

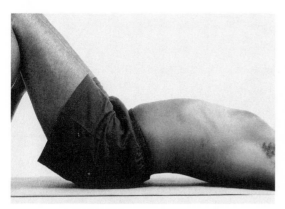 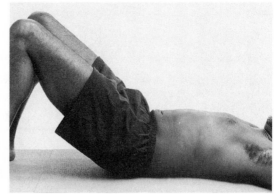

FIG. 19   FIG. 20

DVIPADA PITHAM
Two-Legged Platform or Desk Pose

ABOUT THE POSE: *Dvi* means two. *Pada* is foot. *Pitham* is a platform, table top, or desk. *Dvipada Pitham* facilitates range of motion in the pelvis and the coordination of breath and movement. When we add arm variations, it begins to open both the shoulders and the chest. It is an excellent posture to do at the beginning of a practice to warm up, or at the end of a session as part of a completion sequence leading into final relaxation. Note that we are purposely keeping the spine straight in this version. Sometimes this pose is done as a gentle backbend, similar to Bridge Pose (see Setu Bandhasana).

LET'S PRACTICE

PRELIMINARY MOVEMENT: First perform the "pelvic rock/tilt" several times: Inhale, release the tailbone down toward the floor, slightly lifting the back of the waist off the floor. (Figure 19.) Exhale, drop the navel down and curl the tailbone up, pressing the waistband to the floor. This last movement may also be referred to as a pelvic tilt and is the same as tucking under when you are standing upright. (Figure 20.)

TECHNIQUE: Take a deep breath in and on an exhale, peel the spine off the floor one vertebra at a time, moving slowly to really feel the control of the movement. Once the hips are up, hold your pose and continue breathing slow, rhythmic breaths. (Figure 21.) Do not flare the ribs or puff the chest. There should be a straight slanted line from the knees to the shoulders; with the tailbone and pubic bone higher than the navel, and the navel higher than the sternum. Slightly tighten

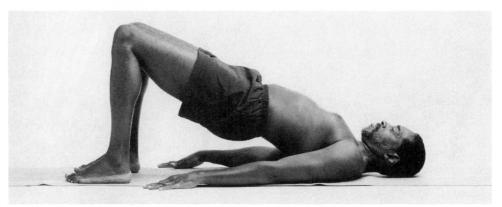

FIG. 21

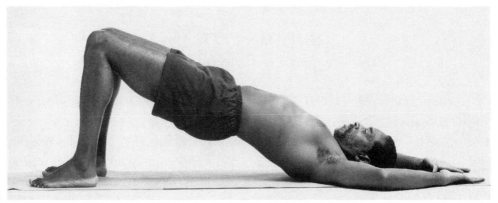

FIG. 22

the buttocks or "tweeze your sit bones," feeling a contraction in the hamstrings, but keep your toes soft and planted on the floor. When you're ready, exhale as you slowly lower the spine down, one vertebra at a time.

VARIATION: ARMS OVERHEAD. Once you feel confident with the pose itself, add the arms. First, in your Basic Supine, bring the arms overhead on the floor, with the elbows bent, on either side of your head, palms facing up. Hold for a few breaths, feeling the opening in the shoulders and the chest without disturbing the alignment of the rest of the spine. Add the "pelvic rock/tilt" from the preliminary movement. Then, keeping the arms overhead, peel the spine off the floor and return to the pose itself. (Figure 22.)

REPETITIONS: Repeat each stage 3 to 5 times.

PREPARATION FOR: *Setu Bandhasana* (Bridge Pose).

BENEFITS: Increases flexibility in the spine, relieves minor lower back discomfort, promotes relaxation.

APANASANA
Knee-to-Chest Pose

ABOUT THE POSE: Since *apana,* Sanskrit for "descending breath," is associated with the lower body and the exhalation, this pose focuses our attention from the waist downward, influencing all of the functions of apana: digestion, assimilation, elimination, and sexual health. Initially you may want to do this pose in a passive or gentle manner. However, it's possible to make it quite an active, or even intense stretch! The Choudhury system refers to this pose as *Pavanamuktasana,* which means "wind-relieving pose." Note that we are adding some additional moves to the standard performance of this pose by including an opening of the knee to side, a supine twist, and an abdominal curl.

LET'S PRACTICE

TECHNIQUE: Take a breath in. Exhale, bringing your right thigh toward your chest. Take hold of your leg by clasping the hands on the top part of the shin or underneath the knee. Chin points down toward the chest. Straighten the left leg on the floor, flexing the foot, pressing out through the heel and contracting the top of the thigh. (Figure 23.) If you can, tighten the fold by clasping the forearms, as though you're giving your knee a hug. Hold here for several breaths.

VARIATION 1: OPENING KNEE TO THE SIDE.

TECHNIQUE: Bring the left arm out to the left at shoulder level, palm facing down, fingers spread. Take hold of the outside of the right knee with your right hand. Inhale. Exhale, opening the right knee out to the side. (Figure 24.) Keep

FIG. 23

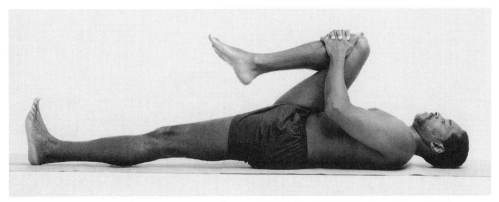

the left buttock in contact with the floor. Lift the chest. The back of the waist may lift slightly from the floor. At the same time, maintain the feeling of tucking under. Most importantly, keep the hips squared toward the ceiling. Continue to press through the left leg and foot. Hold here for a few breaths. Exhale as you lift the knee to the center.

VARIATION 2: SUPINE TWIST.

TECHNIQUE: Inhale, switch arms, bringing the right arm out to the side at shoulder level, palm flat on the floor. Take hold of the right knee with the left hand. Exhale, bring the right knee across the left leg, lifting the right buttock off the floor, and rolling onto the side of the left hip. (Figure 25.) Relax the bottom foot and keep both shoulder blades on the floor. Look to your right, breathe, and hold. Exhale and bring the thigh center. Pause here.

VARIATION 3: ABDOMINAL CURL.

TECHNIQUE: Inhale; clasp the hands around or under the right knee. Exhale, roll the head, neck, and upper back up, drawing your forehead toward your knee. (Figure 26.) Keep elbows spread wide, shoulders down from your earlobes, and the

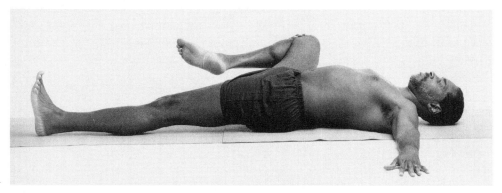

FIG. 24

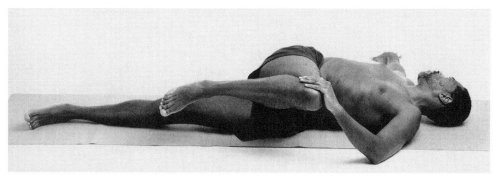

FIG. 25

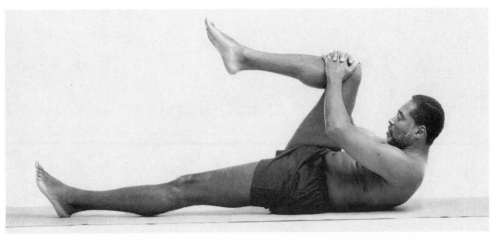

FIG. 26

toes of both feet softly pointed. Keep the left heel on the floor. Hold in this abdominal curl position for 3 to 5 breaths. Inhale, releasing your torso back to the floor. On an exhale, let go of the leg and straighten it down to the floor. Pause here for a few breaths. Repeat on the left side.

REPETITIONS: Repeat entire sequence on both sides once or twice.

PREPARATION FOR: *Supta Padangusthasana* (Supine Leg Stretch).

BENEFITS: Facilitates range of motion in the hip joints, stretches the lower back, lengthens the hip flexors, and tones the abdominals.

SETU BANDHASANA
Bridge Pose

ABOUT THE POSE: *Setu* means a bridge. *Bandha* in this context is the forming of a bridge. In this supine posture, a type of a backbend, the body is arched and supported on the shoulders and feet with arms at your sides or hands clasped underneath your back. In its full form it is a very advanced pose, so we're modifying it for you. At a glance it looks somewhat similar to Dvipada Pitham (Two-Legged Platform Pose), which we give as a preparation for Bridge Pose. In Dvipada Pitham, you keep the spine straight. On the other hand, *Setu Bandhasana* (Bridge Pose) hyperextends, or arches, the spine and requires a good deal of flexibility in the shoulders, chest, and hip flexors. Move slowly into this pose, maintaining the posture at whichever stage is most challenging, yet manageable, for you.

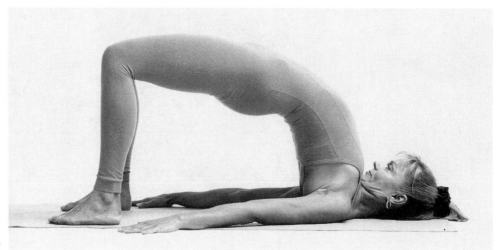

FIG. 27

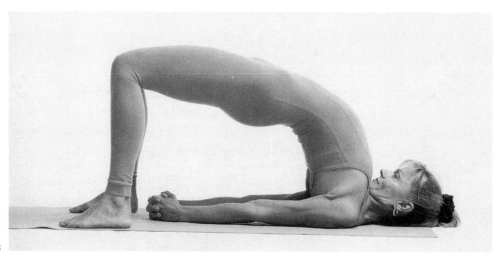

FIG. 28

LET'S PRACTICE

POSITION: Basic Supine, with your feet wider apart than the hips, toes pointing forward, and arms at your sides near your hips with your palms facing down.

TECHNIQUE:

VARIATION 1: Inhale the breath. As you exhale roll the hips up from the floor
leading with the tailbone and pressing into your heels and the balls of your feet
while keeping the toes on the floor. Inhale. Exhale, lift your hips higher, raising
the pubic bone as high as you can. You are now forming an arc, or a bridge.
(Figure 27.) Keep the buttocks very firm, toes on the floor, and the knees in line

with the hips and feet. Hold here and breathe rhythmically for several breaths, keeping your shoulders down and your palms pressing into the floor. Slowly come out of the pose on an exhalation.

VARIATION 2: Move into the pose once again. Keeping the hips lifted, bring your palms together underneath your back. Interlace your fingers, straighten your arms, and press the outer edges of the hands into the floor. Squeeze your shoulder blades together, keep your elbows straight, and reach toward your feet with your hands. (Figure 28.) Hold and breathe for several breaths. When you are ready to come down, inhale, release your hands, and move your arms out from underneath you. Exhale as you slowly lower your back down to the floor.

REPETITIONS: Practice both variations once or twice.

PREPARATION FOR: Backbends and Shoulderstand.

BENEFITS: Increases flexibility in the front body and thighs, while strengthening the back of the body. Stimulating.

CAUTIONS: Even with modifications, Setu Bandhasana is a fairly dynamic and challenging back-bending posture. If you felt as though your back was being pinched while in this pose, its practice may be premature for you at this time. To prepare for this posture, continue to perform Standing Cobra, Two-Legged Platform, Cobra Pose, and the Heel-to-Buttock One-Legged Balance.

APANASANA
Both-Knees-to-Chest Pose

ABOUT THE POSE: This additional variation of Apanasana works well after a backbend like Setu Bandhasana. Pulling both legs toward your chest massages the abdominal organs and stretches out the lower back.

LET'S PRACTICE

TECHNIQUE: Inhale. On an exhale, bring the right knee toward your chest, and then the left knee. Wrap your arms around both your knees and hug them to you. (Figure 29.) Hold here for several breaths. Now, cup the palms of your hands lightly over your kneecaps. Inhaling, draw the knees away from you, straightening the elbows. (Figure 30.) On the exhale, bring the knees toward your chest, curling the tailbone up from the floor, guiding the movement with your hands. (Figure 31.)

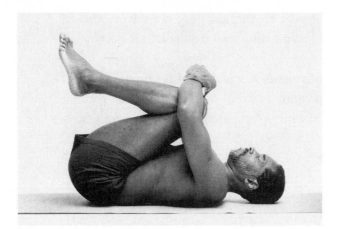

FIG. 29

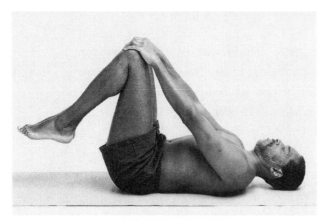

FIG. 30

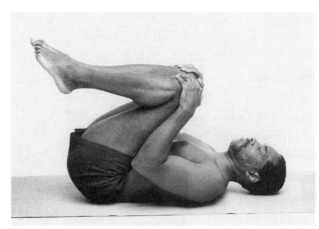

FIG. 31

REPETITIONS: Practice drawing the knees away from you and bringing them into your chest 3 to 5 times.

BENEFITS: Increases blood flow to the abdominal region and the lower back. Aids digestion and elimination.

SUPTA PADANGUSTHASANA
Supine Leg Stretch

ABOUT THE POSE: *Supta* means to be supine, *pada* is foot, and *angustha* is the big toe. A reclining stretch, in this pose you take hold of the big toe and stretch the leg up and to the side. Classically, this posture is done in three stages and includes an abdominal curl. We suggest you use a strap to accommodate tight hamstrings. Of course, if you can hold the big toe with your hand without difficulty, do so. Practice the leg stretch series after you are very warmed up.

LET'S PRACTICE

TECHNIQUE:

Stage 1: Take hold of your strap, placing an end in each hand. Draw the right knee toward you and place your strap over the bottom of the right foot. Relax the shoulders and keep the elbows slightly bent. Inhale the breath and as you exhale press through your heel, firm the thigh, straighten the knee, and flex the foot. Slowly straighten the left leg onto the floor pressing out through the inner seam of that leg and flexing the foot. (Figure 32.) Relax the back into the floor and gently lift the chest. Hold here for several breaths.

Stage 2: With both ends of the strap in the right hand, bring your left arm out to the side at shoulder level, palm pressing down into the floor. Keep your left leg out, stretched on the floor. Inhale as you rotate the right leg out from the hip

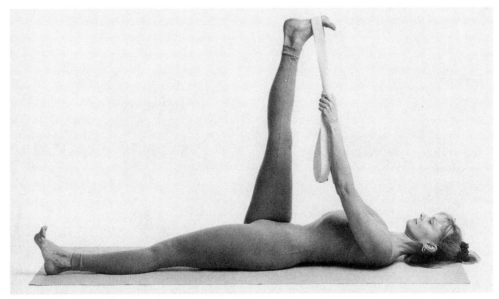

FIG. 32

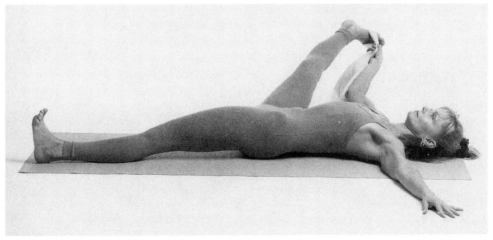

FIG. 33

joint, toes pointing to the side. Exhale and bring the leg toward the right as you turn your head to the left or keep it center. (Figure 33.) Keep the left buttock on the floor and continue to press through the left heel. Inhale. Exhale as you raise the leg back to center.

Stage 3: Inhaling, take hold of both ends of the strap with the left hand and bring your right arm out to the right at shoulder level, palm pressing into the floor. Exhale. Rotate the right leg in and reach it over toward the left as you look toward the right. (Figure 34.) If you need to, bend your right knee a little. The right buttock lifts up. As you roll onto the side of the left hip allow the left foot to relax. Hold for several breaths. Exhale as you return to center.

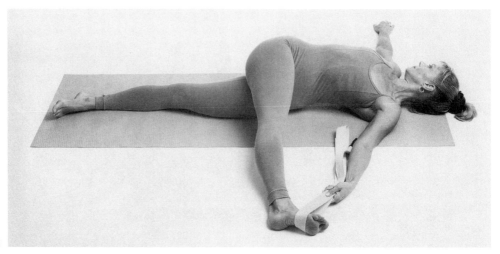

FIG. 34

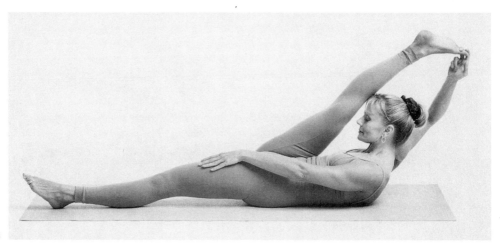

FIG. 35

Stage 4: Once again take hold of both ends of the strap with the right hand. Place your left hand on your left thigh. Inhale the breath. As you exhale curl your head, neck, shoulders, and upper back up from the floor, stretching your left fingertips toward your left knee. As you hold this position decrease the distance between your head and your right leg. Focus on breathing into the sides of the ribs with each inhalation. On your exhalations draw your navel toward your backbone emphasizing the lower abdominal contraction. Hold here for 3 to 5 breaths. To come down, inhale and release your head down to the floor. Exhale as you bend your right leg and release the strap. Lengthen the right leg onto the floor. When you are ready proceed to the left side following all of the above directions.

NOTE: If you feel sufficiently warmed up and flexible, do Stage 4 without a strap, holding the big toe with the index and middle fingers between the big and second toe, closing the thumb around the outside of the big toe. (Figure 35.)

REPETITIONS: One set on both sides is sufficient.

PREPARATION FOR: Standing and seated postures requiring flexibility in the hips and hamstrings.

BENEFITS: Facilitates range of motion in the hip joints; increases flexibility in the hamstrings, the inner thighs (adductors), and the outer thighs (abductors).

CAUTIONS: Not generally recommended for those suffering from sciatica because of the intense stretch in the hamstrings.

7

Prone Poses

The next set of poses are called prone postures, which promote both flexibility and strength in the arms and back. The base position for most of these poses is what we call "Basic Prone." (Figure 36.) Kneeling on all fours, place your hands directly underneath your shoulders and your knees underneath your hips. The spine remains in neutral. Your hands should be flat with fingers spread and the middle fingers pointing forward. Drop your shoulders away from your earlobes; keep the back of the neck long and your face looking at the floor. You're ready to practice.

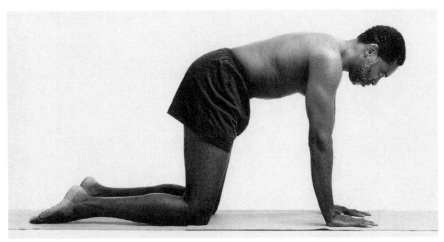

FIG. 36

CHAKRAVAKASANA
The Sunbird (Cat Stretch)

ABOUT THE POSE: Also called "The Ruddy Goose," this basic prone posture is often referred to as "The Cat" or "The Cow." Similar in mechanics to the pelvic rock/tilt which initiated the Two-Legged Platform, this posture provides you with another opportunity to experience range of motion of the spine and the placement of the pelvis. Because you are on your hands and knees this is considered a weight-bearing pose and thus initiates the strengthening of your arms. This pose figures prominently in the Viniyoga tradition.

LET'S PRACTICE

TECHNIQUE: On an inhale, lift your chin and tailbone up, arching the spine. (Figure 37.) You are making a saddle in your back. As you exhale, round your spine, lifting your navel up while moving your head and tailbone down. (Figure 38.) Repeat several times. On your last repetition, inhale and maintain the arch or concave spine. Hold and breathe. Draw your shoulders down from your earlobes, keeping your elbows straight. Exhale as you round the spine with your head and tail down. Hold here and breathe. Separate the shoulder blades. The head is hanging with the neck relaxed. Facial muscles and the throat are soft or passive. When you are ready to release, inhale the breath and return to neutral.

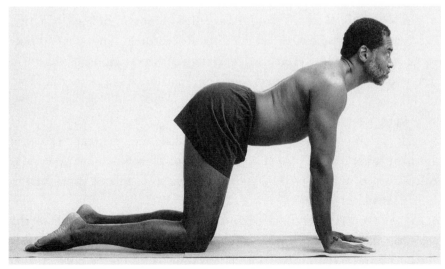

FIG. 37

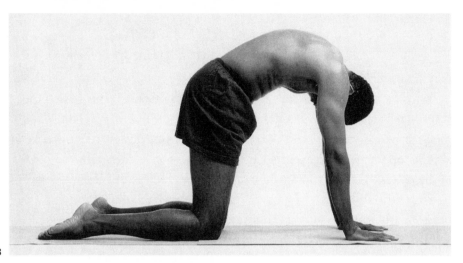

FIG. 38

REPETITIONS: Repeat as often as you like throughout your practice.

PREPARATION FOR: Downward-Facing Dog Pose.

BENEFITS: Creates flexibility in the pelvis and spine; builds strength in the arms.

BALASANA
Child's Pose

ABOUT THE POSE: *Bala* means child. Also called "Embryo" or "Folded Leaf," this is an excellent resting pose to do after a difficult posture or following a backbend. The first variation, "Half-Tortoise," encourages the extension of the torso and arms; the second variation, "Pregnant Tortoise," encourages the abdominals to relax.

LET'S PRACTICE

TECHNIQUE: From your Basic Prone position, inhale the breath and exhaling pull your buttocks back toward your heels. Bring your arms around to your sides with the palms turned upward. Allow your shoulders to drop and your arms to remain totally passive. (Figure 39.)

VARIATION 1: "HALF-TORTOISE." From Basic Prone position, inhale the breath. Exhale as you bring your hips back to rest on your heels. Keep your arms stretched forward. Spread your fingers and flatten your palms on the floor. As you straighten your elbows and pull your shoulders away from your ears, stretch from your fingertips all the way back through your hips. (Figure 40.)

VARIATION 2: "PREGNANT TORTOISE." From Basic Prone, bring the big toes together and separate the knees wider than hips. Inhale and arch the spine, releasing the abdomen toward the floor. As you exhale, draw the buttocks back toward your heels. Fold your arms in front of you and lower the forehead onto them. (Figure 41.)

REPETITIONS: Hold each variation for several breaths. Do this pose as often as you like.

BENEFITS: Brings circulation to the lower back and abdominals, stimulates the organs of the pelvic area, relieves lower back tension.

CAUTIONS: If your knees feel uncomfortable, place a blanket underneath them.

CHATURANGA DANDASANA
Four-Limbed Staff (Plank) Pose

ABOUT THE POSE: In Sanskrit, *chat* is the number four, *anga* means limb, and *danda* is a staff or rod. Similar to the Western-style push-up, Four-Limbed Staff Pose teaches you the importance of proper placement and body mechanics. An advanced pose, *Chaturanga* is part of

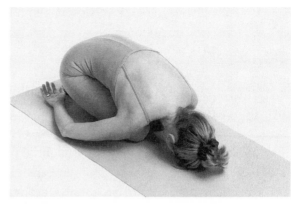

FIG. 39

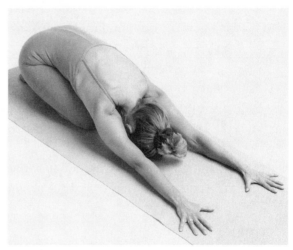

FIG. 40

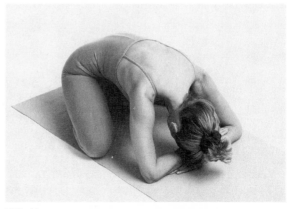

FIG. 41

the Ashtanga yoga version of the jumping Sun Salutation. We are presenting it here in three stages.

LET'S PRACTICE

TECHNIQUE:

Stage 1: Beginning in Basic Prone, bring your hands in front of your shoulders, a full hand space, pointing your center fingers forward. Inhale. On an exhale, bring your hips forward tucking the tail under. Keep your shoulders above your wrists and your elbows straight. From your slanted line, tuck your toes under, inhale the breath, and on an exhale, lift your knees from the floor, pressing into your heels. Again, maintain a straight line from the crown of your head to your tailbone and from your hips to your heels. (Figure 42.) The buttocks should stay very firm while you maintain a pelvic tilt. *Do not allow the back to collapse.* (Figure 43—incorrect.) Hold for a couple of breaths. Inhale and lower your knees. Exhale as you bring your hips back to Half-Tortoise and rest.

Stage 2: Lie flat on your stomach. Bend your elbows and bring them close to your rib cage. Place your hands flat on the floor, fingers spread, middle fingers pointing forward. Feet should be hip-distance apart. Inhaling, turn your head to face the floor, tuck your toes under, and flex the feet. On an exhale, press into your forearms and lift yourself into a horizontal position. Keep the elbows on the floor, maintain the pelvic tilt, and firm the buttocks and thighs. Continue to look down at the floor as you draw your shoulders away from your earlobes, and lengthen

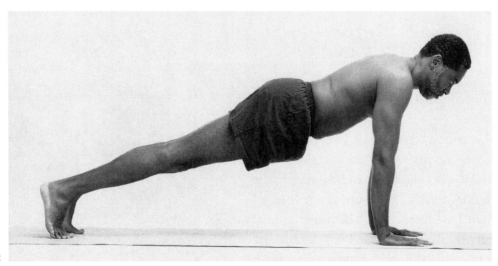

FIG. 42

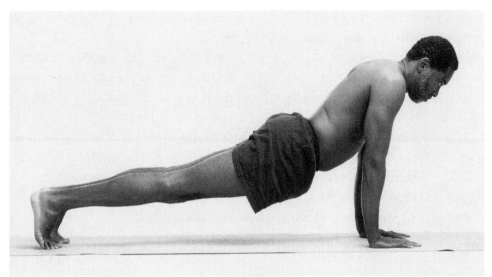

FIG. 43
(INCORRECT)

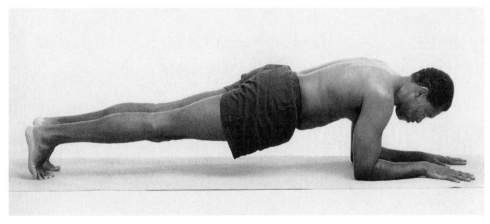

FIG. 44

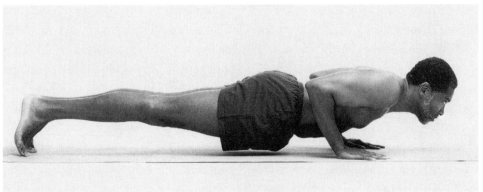

FIG. 45

through your neck. (Figure 44.) Hold for a few breaths. Release to the floor. Relax your arms and legs and turn your head to the side.

Stage 3: The Classic Pose. Place your hands directly underneath your shoulders, with fingers spread and middle fingers pointing forward. Bend the elbows and press them into your ribs. Place the feet hip-distance apart, flex them, and tuck the toes under. Look forward, drawing your chin away from the base of the throat. Inhale. Exhale, pressing up from the floor just a couple of inches. Keep the tailbone tucked and the abdominals lifted. (Figure 45.) Hold for one or two breaths. Lower down on the exhalation. Turn your head to the side and relax completely.

REPETITIONS: Practice each stage twice.

BENEFITS: Strengthens the arms, legs, and abdominals.

CAUTIONS: For students with weak abdominals, Stages 2 and 3 may prove too challenging. Practice Stage 1 instead, and strengthen the abdominals by doing Twisted Stomach Pose and Full Boat Pose.

BHUJANGASANA
Cobra Pose

ABOUT THE POSE: *Bhujanga* is a serpent. This posture, commonly called Cobra Pose, shows up in virtually every style of hatha yoga in one form or another. Here are two stages of the pose—a very modified beginner's version and the final, classic, form of *Bhujangasana*—plus a modified version of the classic pose.

LET'S PRACTICE

TECHNIQUE:

Stage 1: The Sphinx. Lie on your stomach. Bend your elbows and place them directly under the shoulders. Place your forearms on the floor, parallel to one another; hands are flat, fingers spread with middle fingers pointing forward. Shoulders are down from the earlobes and the legs are hip-distance apart. Looking forward a few inches beyond the line of the fingertips, lift the chest and shoulders from the floor. Relax your throat and facial muscles and firm the buttocks and thighs. The toes remain on the floor. Hold and breathe for a few breaths. Release. (Figure 46.)

Stage 2: The Classic Pose. Bend your elbows and place your hands directly underneath your shoulders. Draw the legs together, with the inner thighs, knees, and heels actively touching. With the back of your neck lengthening, gaze toward

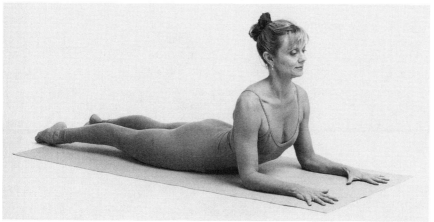

FIG. 46

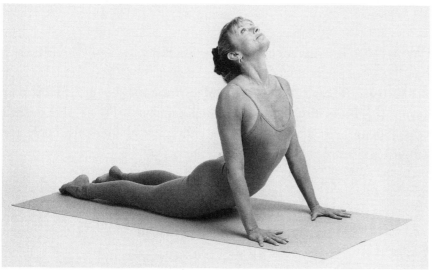

FIG. 47

the floor in front of you. Press your pubic bone down as you draw your buttocks together and tighten the thighs. Inhale and begin to lift the chest up and chin forward. Keep your toes on the floor. Exhale. Inhaling, lift the chest a few degrees higher, shifting part of your weight onto your arms. Hold here and exhale. As you lift one more time through the chest, straighten your arms. Keeping the shoulders down, bring the head farther back and either keep the eyes open, or inwardly gaze at the "third eye," the point between the eyebrows. (Figure 47.) Hold for a few breaths. When you are ready, release your chin forward. Inhale. Exhale, releasing to the floor.

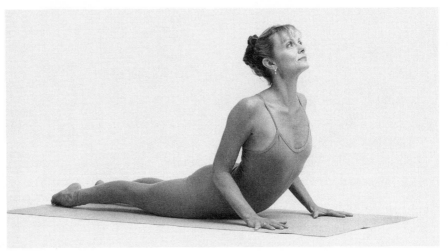

FIG. 48

REPETITIONS: Do both stages once or twice, or repeat a single variation two or three times.

MODIFICATIONS: If Stage 2 is too much of a stretch for you, modify the pose by keeping your legs hip-width apart and your elbows bent. (Figure 48.)

BENEFITS: Strengthens the back muscles, arms, and abdominals; opens the chest and improves posture.

ADHO MUKHA SVANASANA
Downward-Facing Dog Pose

ABOUT THE POSE: *Adho* means down, *mukha* means face, and *svana* is a dog. This weight-bearing posterior stretch is a perennial favorite of Iyengar instructors and plays an integral part in both the Classic- and the Ashtanga-style Sun Salutations. It requires a certain amount of flexibility in the shoulder joints and the chest, as well as the pelvis and legs.

LET'S PRACTICE

PREPARATORY MOVEMENT: Place your hands flat on the wall 6 to 10 inches above hip level. Step back from the wall, straightening your elbows and flattening your back. Your feet should be hip-distance apart and your toes should point forward. (Figure 49.) Keep the neck in line with your arms and look toward the floor. If you can straighten your legs, contract the thighs and lift your kneecaps. If

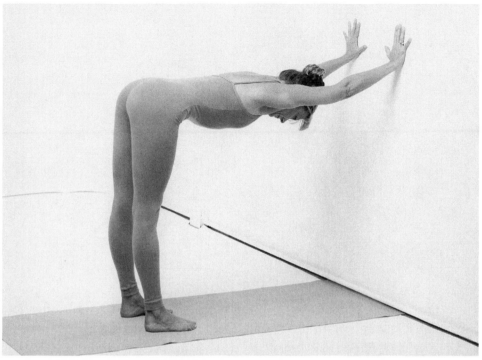

FIG. 49

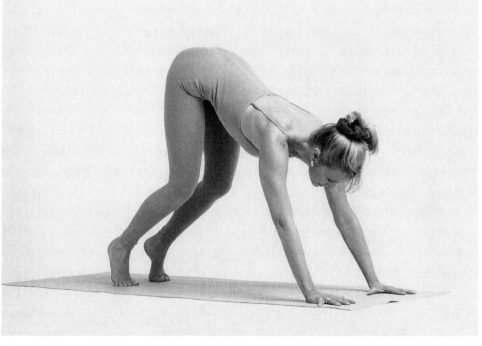

FIG. 50

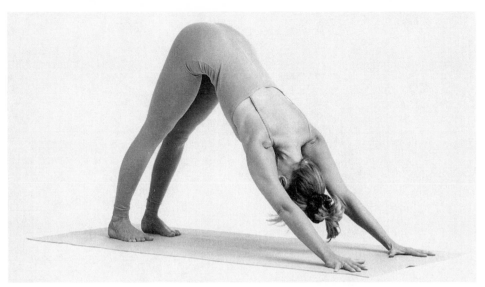

FIG. 51

your hamstrings are really tight, keep the knees bent and focus on releasing your tailbone back and up toward the ceiling. Hold for several breaths.

TECHNIQUE: From Basic Prone, gently arch the back, with the chin and tail up. Tuck your toes under, flexing the feet. Inhale the breath. On an exhale, point the tailbone up toward the ceiling and raise your knees off the floor. With your heels raised and your knees bent, press your chest back toward your thighs. (Figure 50.) On another inhale, straighten your knees and lift your hips even higher. Exhale and lower your heels to the floor. Allow your head to relax in between your arms, keeping the throat and face relaxed. Contract the front of the thighs and lift your kneecaps. At the same time, release downward through the backs of your legs, pressing into your heels. (Figure 51.) Maintain this posture for 3 to 5 breaths. When you are ready to come down, inhale and raise your heels up. Exhale as you lower to your knees. Inhale and release your feet. Exhale as you pull your buttocks back toward your heels.

REPETITIONS: Practice this 2 or 3 times.

BENEFITS: Stretches the hamstrings and calf muscles, creates traction in the spine, tones the abdominals, strengthens the arms and wrists, and opens up the shoulders and the chest.

CAUTIONS: Stiffness in the upper back, shoulders, and chest may prevent you from moving far enough into the pose to experience a good hamstring stretch. If so, practice the preparatory movement instead.

8

Standing Poses

Now we begin the more dynamic part of your practice. The following sequences will provide you with a core repertoire of standing poses particularly good for strength and balance. Mountain Pose (*Tadasana*) begins and ends all of your standing postures. Consider it your "Basic Stance."

TADASANA
Mountain Pose

ABOUT THE POSE: *Tada* means mountain. Also referred to as *samasthiti,* which means pose of balance, *Tadasana* will begin and end all your standing poses. The practice of this pose establishes the fundamentals of placement and alignment, the principles of which will be carried out in all standing poses. The emphasis in this posture is on creating a foundation of stability and symmetry. This pose is common in all styles of hatha yoga.

LET'S PRACTICE

TECHNIQUE: Stand with your feet together, toes pointing forward and arms at your sides. Relax your shoulders; keep your chin parallel to the floor. The big toes should touch, with the heels slightly apart and the outer edges of the feet parallel to one another. (Figures 52 and 53.) Your body weight should be evenly distributed between the toes and heels and from right to left. To straighten your legs,

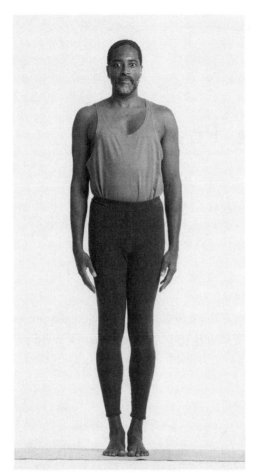

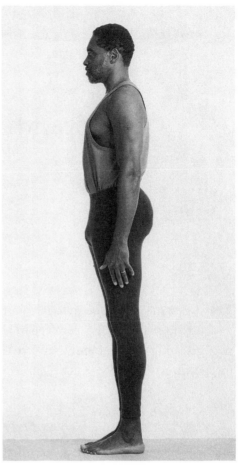

FIG. 52   FIG. 53

contract your thighs, which will lift your kneecaps. Firm the buttocks and keep the pelvis in neutral position as you draw the abdominals in and up and lift your chest. Drop your shoulders away from your earlobes, lower your chin slightly, and keep your throat soft. Lengthen the back of the neck, lifting into the crown of the head.

REPETITIONS: Hold for several breaths, breathing rhythmically. Since this posture is done in between all other standing poses, you'll have ample opportunity to practice it.

IMAGE: The image of a mountain is most obvious. Cultivate the feelings of being solid and tall. Have a sense of rooting your feet into the earth, while growing heavenward through the top of your head.

BENEFITS: Improves posture, builds strength, and develops stamina; key elements necessary to performing all standing poses.

CAUTIONS: If you are uncomfortable with your feet so close together, separate them a little as they do in the Viniyoga tradition. If keeping your knees straight puts pressure on your knees or lower back, bend them slightly.

ARDHA CHANDRASANA
Half-Moon Pose

ABOUT THE POSE: *Ardha* means half, and *chandra* is moon. The Half-Moon Pose addresses lateral flexion of the spine and is preparatory to all sideward bending postures. This particular variation is Bikram Choudhury's Half-Moon posture. The Iyengar Half-Moon Pose is far more advanced and involves a one-leg balance. Although the Choudhury Half-Moon is very simple to do mechanically, it is nonetheless an intense stretch. A less intense version of this pose appears in the Breathing Exercises section.

LET'S PRACTICE

BASE POSITION: Tadasana.

TECHNIQUE: As you inhale, rotate your palms out and bring your arms up overhead. Touching your fingers together, cross one thumb over the other. Take another couple of breaths here, as you extend through your arms. Straighten your elbows as firmly as you can, keeping the arms aligned with your plumb line. (Figure 54.) The throat and neck remain relaxed. Keep your eyes open, gazing straight ahead.

Inhale, stretching tall. On an exhale, stretch directly to your right, hips pressing toward the left, lengthening the underneath side of the rib cage as

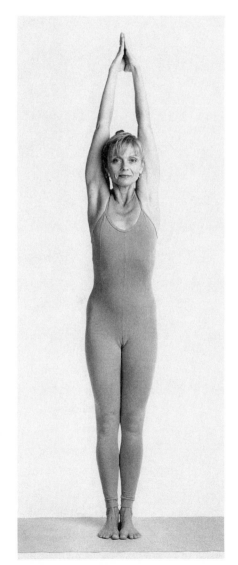

FIG. 54

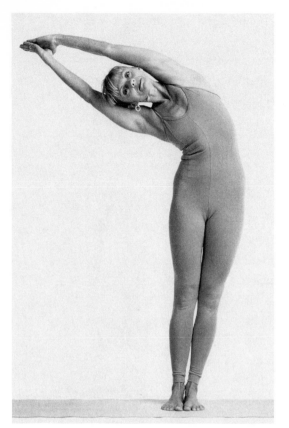

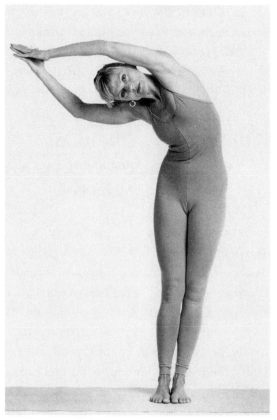

FIG. 55   FIG. 56 (INCORRECT)

much as possible. (Figure 55.) *Take care not to twist in the waist or bend forward.* (Figure 56—incorrect.) Hold here and breathe. Inhale to come up. Repeat on the left side. On an inhale, return to center. Pause there and exhale, stretching up again. On an exhale, open your arms down to your sides, completing the pose.

REPETITIONS: Repeat once or twice.

FOCUS: Half-Moon Pose teaches you how to remain on the same plane or bend directly to the side, without torquing or bending forward. This develops your proprioceptive awareness, the sensing of how your body is placed and moves in space.

BENEFITS: Strengthens the legs and the musculature of the torso, encourages flexibility of the shoulder joints, and tones the arm muscles. This pose also has a positive effect on the kidneys, liver, spleen, and the digestive system. It's an excellent pose in preparation for twists.

COUNTERPOSE: Forward bends and backbends.

CAUTIONS: If the shoulder joints are tight, or your lower back is sensitive, substitute the Modified Half-Moon on page 58.

UTKATASANA
Chair Pose

ABOUT THE POSE: *Utkata* means powerful and fierce, as well as awkward and uneven. Because it looks and feels like you're sitting in a chair, this posture is often referred to as Chair Pose. Although there are several variations of this posture, we'll introduce you to two of them, both excellent postures for building strength and stamina. We've also included a modified version at the wall.

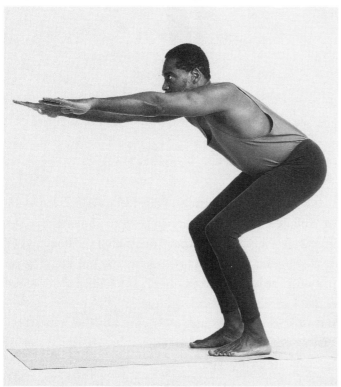

FIG. 57

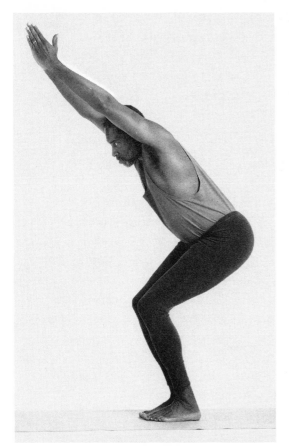

FIG. 58

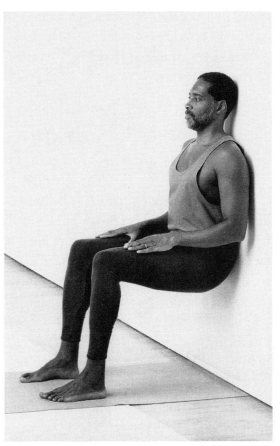

FIG. 59

LET'S PRACTICE

TECHNIQUE:

VARIATION 1: CHOUDHURY-STYLE. Stand with your feet parallel to one another, about 6 inches apart. Inhale and bring your arms up to shoulder height, shoulder distance apart. Fingers are together with the palms facing the floor and elbows straight. Exhale and release your hips back as though you are going to sit down. Keep the knees in line with the hips and toes, the chest lifted, and the shoulders away from the earlobes. Look straight forward. (Figure 57.) To come out of the pose, inhale and straighten your knees. Exhale and lower your arms to your sides.

VARIATION 2: IYENGAR-STYLE. Bring feet together. On an inhale, bring your arms out to shoulder level, rotating your palms to face upward. Exhale. Inhale and continue lifting your arms up overhead, touching your palms together without crossing any of your fingers. Straighten your elbows, feeling your inner arms against your ears and head. Keep your throat soft and shoulders away from your earlobes. Exhaling, release your buttocks back. Bend your knees, bringing your thighs as close as you can to a horizontal alignment while keeping the heels on the floor. The chest will release forward to some degree; however, attempt to keep the shoulders above the hips. (Figure 58.)

REPETITIONS: Hold either of these variations for 3 to 5 breaths. Repeat each one 2 or 3 times. If you practice both in one session, begin with the first variation.

MODIFICATIONS: Practice at the wall. The back should stay flat against the wall, with your feet far enough forward so that the knees are over the ankles, the shins perpendicular, and the thighs parallel to the floor. Hold the arms out in front of you, as in variation 1, or place your hands on your thighs. (Figure 59.) To modify variation 2, keep the arms apart and in line with the shoulders, or even wider.

FOCUS: On the back of the body: the hamstrings and buttocks.

BENEFITS: Strengthens the back and the legs and tones the arms. The Iyengar variation also relieves stiffness in the shoulder joints.

COUNTERPOSE: Forward-bending poses, such as Uttanasana, to extend and stretch the hamstrings.

CAUTIONS: Although this pose is excellent for strengthening the thighs, it can aggravate knee problems if performed incorrectly. Keep the knees tracked correctly, maintaining the congruent hip, knee, and ankle alignment in both variations.

UTTANASANA
Forward Bend

ABOUT THE POSE: *Ut* indicates deliberation or intensity. *Tan* is to stretch, extend, or lengthen out. One of the most basic of the standing forward-bending postures, *Uttanasana* is a deliberate and intense stretch of the hamstrings that shows up in most styles of hatha yoga. Understanding this posture and performing it in good form will establish the proper body mechanics of all forward-bending poses.

LET'S PRACTICE

TECHNIQUE: With feet together, inhale the breath. As you exhale, release back through the buttocks, bringing your torso over your thighs. Place your hands

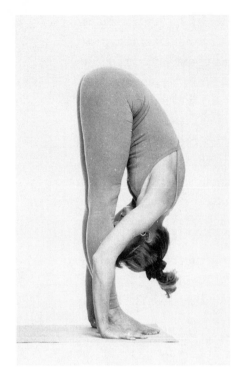

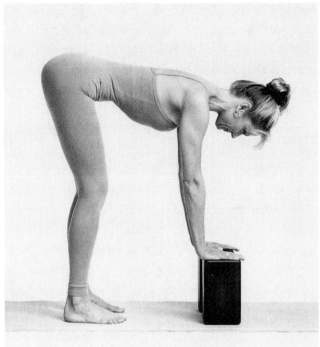

FIG. 60   FIG. 61

on the floor. Keep the knees very straight by contracting the thighs; place the hands outside the feet with palms pressing into the floor. Initially, keep the head up, drawing the sternum away from the pubic bone and the tailbone away from the navel. Hold and breathe for a few breaths. Shift your weight slightly toward your toes without gripping them. Exhale the breath as you draw your head down and in toward your knees. (Figure 60.) Keep your shoulders and throat soft. When you are ready to come up, inhale and lift your head. Keeping your head up, on your next exhale, bring the hands to the hips as you lift the torso to the horizontal alignment. Finally inhale and lift upright. Exhale as you release your arms to your sides.

REPETITIONS: Because this is such an intense stretch, it is best to move into and out of it slowly. Practice it 2 or 3 times in succession, relaxing in between your efforts.

MODIFICATIONS: To accommodate very tight hamstrings and inflexibility in the lower back, we recommend that you use blocks. Place the blocks 12 to 15 inches out in front of your toes. With feet parallel and hip-distance apart, bend your knees slightly and release your hips back. Lean forward, keeping the spine long. Inhale, and place your hands flat on top of the blocks. (Figure 61.) Exhale and draw your navel up to your spine, keeping your back flat. When you are ready to come up, bend your knees slightly more, place your hands on your hips, inhale, and come upright. Exhale and relax your arms to your sides.

FOCUS: On the extension of the hamstrings and the lengthening of the spine.

BENEFITS: Stretches the hamstrings, extends the spine, and strengthens the back muscles. This pose has a calming effect on the system.

CAUTIONS: If you have a history of sciatica, you will need to approach this pose—and all postures involving forward flexion—cautiously.

THE HINDI SQUAT

ABOUT THE POSE: A common position practiced by East Indians on a daily basis, the Hindi Squat is not technically a yoga pose, but rather the foundation of several classic postures. Although most of us squatted as infants and young children, we lose this natural ability as we grow older. The Hindi Squat particularly affects the lower back and pelvic area as well as hip, knee, and ankle joints. Even though this is a deep knee bend, your body weight will be centered in the pelvic area—not over the knees—so that the feet can stay flat on the floor with the heels down. Therefore, this pose is **not** bad for your knees. However, if you've had problems with either your hips or knees, proceed cautiously. In most cases, it is tightness in the lower back or hips that will prevent you from doing this pose.

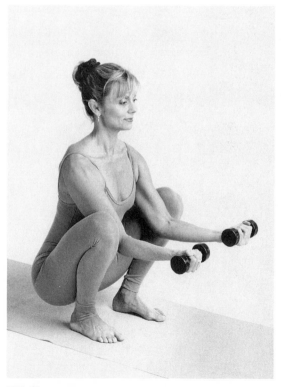

FIG. 62

LET'S PRACTICE

TECHNIQUE:

VARIATION 1: WITH WEIGHTS. Use two one- to two-pound dumbbells, two 16-ounce soup cans, or a one-liter bottle of water. Either hold a single weight in both hands, or place one weight in each hand. Begin in Basic Stance, feet parallel to one another, shoulder-distance or slightly wider apart, approximately 10–15 inches. Hold the weights from underneath in the palms of your hands. Relax your shoulders and bend your elbows so that the weights stay fairly close to your body. Inhale. As you exhale, bend your knees, releasing your buttocks back, and begin to lower yourself toward the floor. As you do this, reach your weights away from you to the front—about 6–8 inches. This counterbalances the weight of your hips moving back and downward. Keep your heels flat and your knees directly over your toes. (Figure 62.) In the beginning, you may not be able to go all the way to the floor. Go as far as you can. Hold for a few breaths. If you can go all the way down, your buttocks will hover just a few inches above the floor and your knees will open to allow your torso to come forward in between them. Your elbows will be on the insides of your knees. As you hold and breathe, exert pressure between your arms and thighs and lift up through your chest. Exhale as you lift up, engaging your abdominals, thighs, and buttocks.

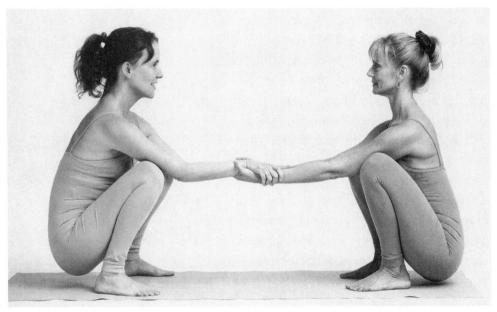

FIG. 63

VARIATION 2: WITH A PARTNER. Face your partner and take hold of one another's wrists. Follow the directions for the first variation. You may need to adjust the distance between you. Hold one another's wrists or hands for the whole exercise. Keep your heels on the floor. When you are down in the squat, your arms will remain on the inside of your knees, and your torsos will be inclined toward one another. (Figure 63.) Hold for several breaths. Come up in unison on an exhalation.

VARIATION 3: FREE STANDING. Follow the directions for the first variation. Begin with your hands on your hips. When you get all the way down, place your hands in a prayer position in front of your chest. Press your knees open with your elbows and lift up through the chest and the crown of your head. (Figure 64.) Hold for several breaths.

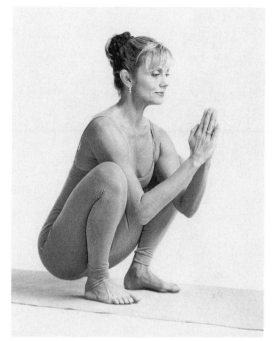

FIG. 64

REPETITIONS: Practice whichever variation works for you 2 or 3 times.

FOCUS: Keep your feet flat, heels down, and the knees tracking over the toes. As much as you can, keep your feet in their original parallel placement.

BENEFITS: Increases flexibility in the lower back, hips, and calves; strengthens the buttocks, hamstrings, and quadriceps; and tones the abdominal area. Excellent for digestion and elimination, and as an antidote for the lower back discomfort from menstruation. Include Hindi Squat in the cooling down stretching sequences you do after aerobic or athletic activity.

COUNTERPOSE: Standing forward-bending poses which stretch the hamstrings, such as Uttanasana or Prasarita Padottanasana, are best.

Expanding Your Stance

The next three poses require a wide stance. We suggest you come into this position from Tadasana in one of two ways—either stepping or jumping your feet wide apart. Practice either of the following techniques as a drill several times. How you move into, and out of, a posture is as important as the pose itself.

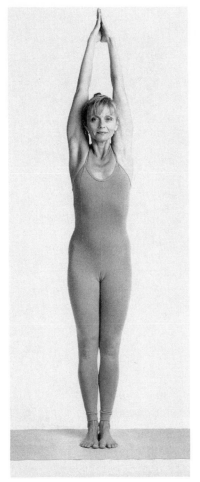

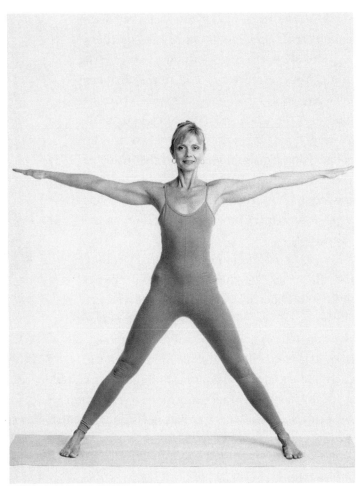

FIG. 65A   FIG. 65B

STEPPING TECHNIQUE: From Tadasana, bring your arms up overhead and place your hands flat together. Inhale and stretch upward into your hands. (Figure 65A.) As you exhale, step the right leg open to a wide stance, both feet facing forward, and bring your arms out to the sides at shoulder level, palms facing down. (Figure 65B.) To return to Tadasana, bring your legs together, pressing from your right foot. Repeat to the left.

JUMPING TECHNIQUE: From Tadasana, bend your knees and bring your hands to your chest, palms facing down and middle fingers touching. Inhale. (Figure 66.) On the exhale, jump your feet apart to a wide stance and spread your arms out to shoulder level, palms facing down. (Figure 67.)

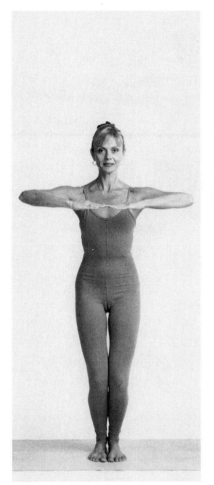

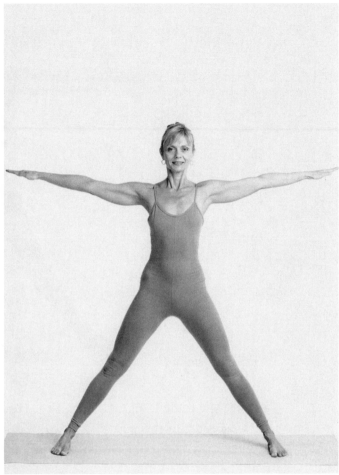

FIG. 66   FIG. 67

When you're ready to go into a posture, adjust the feet and proceed as directed. To complete the pose, turn both feet forward and step, or jump, back to Tadasana.

UTTHITA TRIKONASANA
Triangle Pose

ABOUT THE POSE: *Utthita* means extended, or stretched. *Tri* is three, and *kona* is angle. A lateral stretch, Triangle Pose allows the torso to extend to the side

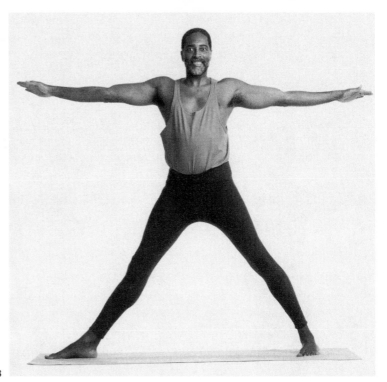

FIG. 68

and over the leading leg. All yoga styles teach *Trikonasana,* although there are many variations of this pose.

PREPARATORY POSTURE (IF NECESSARY): Half-Moon Pose—Choudhury style.

LET'S PRACTICE

BASE POSITION: Your feet are approximately 3 to 3½ feet (or the length of one of your legs) apart. Turn your left foot in 30 degrees and your right foot out 90 degrees. Keep your right heel in line with the arch of your left foot. Your right knee is in line with your right foot. Keep your kneecaps lifted by contracting your thighs. Arms are open at shoulder level, palms facing the floor. (Figure 68.)

TECHNIQUE: Inhale the breath. Exhale and shift your pelvis to the left as you reach out to the right, extending your torso to the side over your right leg. (Figure 69.) Place your right hand on your right shin or ankle. Your left arm is stretched upward in line with the shoulder, palm facing forward. Turn your head so that you can look directly up toward your left thumb. (Figure 70.) Breathe rhythmically. To come out of the pose, turn your head toward your bottom leg, bending that

knee slightly, and inhale as you come upright. Exhale and turn your right foot forward. Relax your arms down to your sides. Keep your legs open, lift your arms,
and proceed to the left. Your right foot will now turn in, and the left foot will turn
out.

REPETITIONS: The pace is moderate. Hold the pose for 3 to 5 breaths. After
doing the pose on both sides, return to Tadasana. Repeat the whole process once
or twice more.

MODIFICATIONS: If you have difficulty balancing, or if you can't reach your
ankle or shin bone, place a block behind your front foot and rest your hand on it.
(Figure 71.) If your hamstrings are really tight, you may want to keep the knee of
the leading leg slightly bent while in this pose. The neck may also be sensitive. If
so, alternately turn the head down and look up again, toward the upper hand, as
you hold this pose.

EMPHASIS: On maintaining the torso in direct lateral alignment or on the
same plane as the legs and hips.

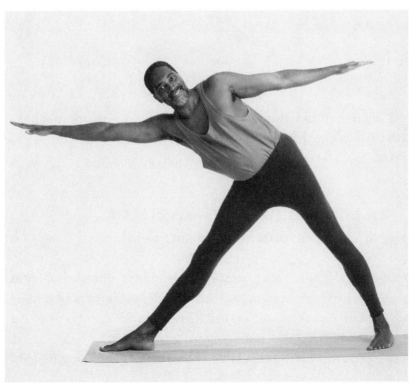

FIG. 69

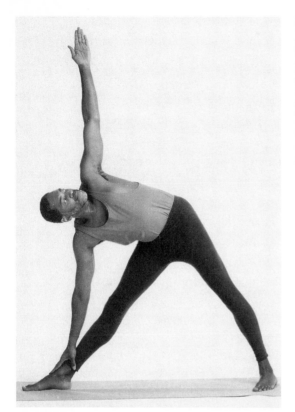

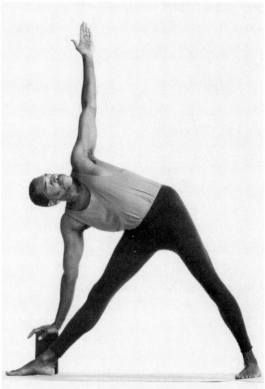

FIG. 70

FIG. 71

BENEFITS: Strengthens the legs and encourages flexibility in the hips. Stretches and strengthens the musculature of the torso.

COUNTERPOSE: Both forward and backward bending postures.

PRASARITA PADOTTANASANA I
Spread Legs Intense Forward Bend

ABOUT THE POSE: *Prasarita* means expanded, spread, or extended. *Pada* is foot. The wide stance taken in this posture will bring your awareness to your inner and outer thighs. It will also allow you greater freedom in the movement of the pelvis as you release the hips back, in order to bend forward.

PREPARATORY POSTURE (IF NECESSARY): Downward-Facing Dog Pose, at the wall.

LET'S PRACTICE

BASE POSITION: Wide stance with feet approximately 4½ to 5 feet apart. Turn your toes in a few degrees, so that your feet are slightly pigeon-toed.

TECHNIQUE: Place your hands on your hips. Inhale the breath and bend slightly backward, keeping the buttocks firm. Exhale and bring the chest forward as you release your tailbone back. Keep your thighs contracted and your kneecaps lifted. Place the hands on the floor, keeping them shoulder-width apart, fingertips in line with the toes. Pause, inhale, and lift the head up as you press down into your hands. Exhale and release the head down toward the floor as you bend your elbows. (Figure 72.) Reach the crown of the head toward the floor. Keep the weight in the legs. At the same time, press through your arms as you extend down through your spine and up through the backs of the legs. When you are ready to come out, place your hands on your hips and bring the spine parallel to the floor. Inhale and come all the way up. Exhale and relax your arms to your sides. Jump, or step, your feet into Tadasana.

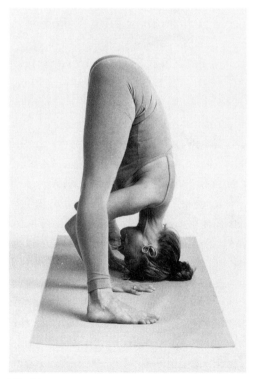

FIG. 72

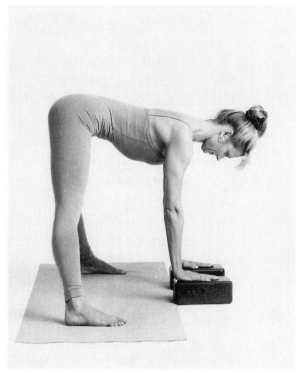

FIG. 73

REPETITIONS: Hold this posture for 3 to 5 breaths. Practice once or twice.

MODIFICATIONS: If the 4½- to 5-foot-spread is too wide for you, bring your feet closer together. If your hands don't reach the floor use blocks to support them. (Figure 73.)

BENEFITS: Strengthens the legs and creates flexibility in the hamstrings.

COUNTERPOSE: Chair Pose or Hindi Squat.

CAUTIONS: If you have a history of sciatica, you will need to approach this pose—and all postures involving forward flexion—cautiously.

UTTHITA PARSVAKONASANA
Side Angle Pose

ABOUT THE POSE: *Utthita* means extended. *Parsva* is a side, or flank. *Kona* is an angle. This is a very dynamic posture which is equally active for both the lower and upper body.

PREPARATORY POSTURE (IF NECESSARY): Half-Moon or Triangle Pose.

LET'S PRACTICE

TECHNIQUE: Your feet are approximately 4 to 4½ feet apart. Turn your right foot out 90 degrees, and your left foot in 30 degrees. Check that your right heel is in line with the arch of your back foot. Keep your kneecaps lifted by contracting your thighs. Arms are open at shoulder level, palms facing the floor.

LEVEL 1: On an exhale, bend your right knee bringing it in line with the ankle, and the shin perpendicular to the floor. Inhale, and on an exhale, reach your torso to the right and take hold of the right calf or ankle with the right hand. Press the right thigh open, or back, with your right forearm. Inhale and extend your left arm open at shoulder level, turning the palm to face the ceiling. As you exhale, bring the arm straight up above the shoulder. (Figure 74.) The palm will face the front of the room. You may either look up at the extended hand or keep your head forward, the neck in line with the angle of the torso. Return to center and proceed to the other side.

LEVEL 2: THE CLASSIC POSE. If necessary, spread the legs wider, turning the right foot out and the left foot in. In this version your right thigh needs to be parallel to the floor and the shin in vertical alignment, the knee above the ankle. Repeat Level 1, but this time place the right arm behind the right leg,

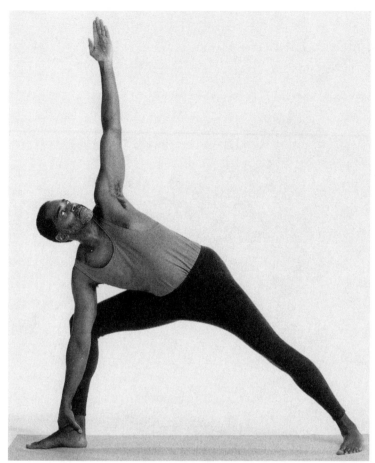

FIG. 74

with the palm flat on the floor. Inhale and rotate the left arm open within the shoulder joint, palm facing the ceiling. As you exhale bring the left arm over the side and overhead without covering your face. Turn the head and look up to the extended hand, the palm of which continues to face the floor. (Figure 75.) Keep the back thigh very firm. Continue to press the right thigh back. Buttocks are firm and abdominals are lifted, maintaining the tuck of the pelvis. When you are ready, come out of the pose on an inhalation. Exhale and turn your right foot forward, releasing your arms down to your sides. Repeat to the other side.

REPETITIONS: Hold each stage for at least 2 to 3 breaths. Repeat either variation once or twice.

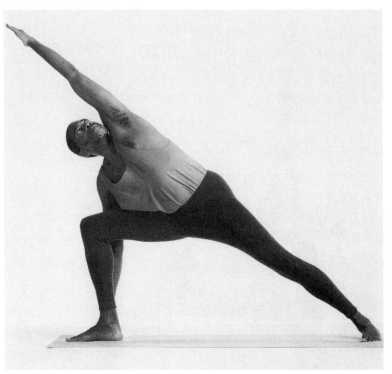

FIG. 75

MODIFICATIONS: Use a block if you need to, placing it behind the foot to support the bottom hand.

EMPHASIS: On extending the torso laterally, while maintaining a strong base in the legs and hips.

BENEFITS: Strengthens the legs and back muscles, tones the waist, opens the hips and shoulders.

COUNTERPOSE: Uttanasana or Prasarita Padottanasana.

9

⧈⧈

Balancing Poses

The one-legged balances in the yoga repertoire offer the opportunity to refine our own balance. The equilibrium we attain by practicing these poses is essential to maintaining the coordination to move comfortably, safely, and effectively throughout our lives.

Although you may practice balances at any time, completing your standing series with a one-legged balance is particularly powerful. Balancing postures represent an integration of the technical elements required of you in all standing poses. We've chosen Tree Pose, a classic balancing asana common to all styles of hatha yoga. To set you up for Tree Pose, we've included a short preparatory sequence.

STANDING KNEE-TO-CHEST

LET'S PRACTICE

TECHNIQUE: Begin in Basic Stance. Choose a point in front of you on which to focus—at eye level or slightly above—and maintain this point throughout the pose. Inhale the breath and shift your weight to your left leg. As you exhale, bend the right knee and bring it up toward your chest. Interlace your fingers just below the kneecap. (Figure 76.) Keep your shoulders down and chest lifted. Elbows are pointing downward. Straighten the standing leg and contract the front of that

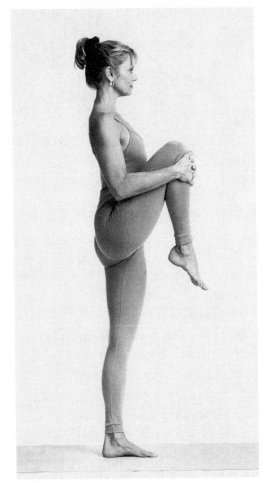

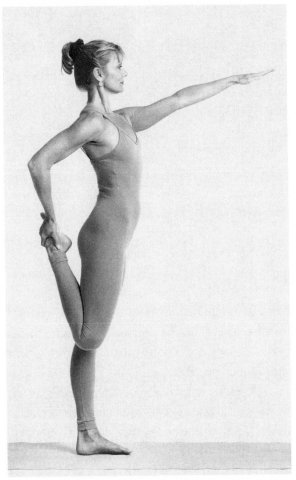

FIG. 76

FIG. 77

thigh, lifting the kneecap. The foot on the floor is flat, with the toes soft and spread. Lift up through the arch, while keeping the big toe joint pressed into the floor. The foot of the lifted leg is passive, toes relaxed downward. Hold for several breaths, breathing rhythmically. When you are ready, release your hands and lower the leg to the floor. Pause in your Basic Stance for a few breaths. Repeat on the other side.

REPETITIONS: Repeat once or twice more.

BENEFITS: Releases tension in the lower back, promotes balance, strengthens the standing leg, and activates the hip flexors.

STANDING HEEL-TO-BUTTOCK

TECHNIQUE: Begin in Basic Stance. Choose a point in front of you on which to focus—at eye level or slightly above—and maintain this point throughout the pose. Inhale the breath and shift your weight to your left leg. As you exhale, bend your right knee, take hold of the top of the right foot or ankle with the right hand, and draw the heel up toward the buttock. Place the left hand on the left hip or raise it straight out in front of you, slightly higher than shoulder level. (Figure 77.) Keep the arm straight and the fingers together. Draw your knees together, bringing your thighs onto the same plane. Tuck the tailbone under and lift your chest. Breathe and hold for several breaths. To come out of the pose, release the foot and lower the upper arm. Bring your arms to your sides. Return to Basic Stance and remain here for a few breaths. Repeat, balancing on your right leg.

REPETITIONS: Repeat the sequence once or twice more.

BENEFITS: In addition to strengthening the legs and developing your balance, this pose stretches the hip flexors and quadriceps. This posture perfectly complements the one before it: While the first one directs the knee up and toward your chest, this pose places the knee down and away from your front body.

VRKSASANA
Tree Pose

ABOUT THE POSE: *Vrksa* is a tree. Tree Pose is the most elementary one-leg balance in the classic hatha yoga repertoire.

LET'S PRACTICE

TECHNIQUE: Inhale and shift your weight to the left leg. Exhaling, bend your right knee and pick up your right ankle with your right hand. From here on, breathe rhythmically. Place the sole of the right foot on the inside of the left thigh, as high up as possible. Place your hands at your heart in what is called the *anjali mudra* or prayer position (Figure 78) or reach your arms up overhead, fingers together and thumbs crossed. (Figure 79.) Keep the standing leg strong, with the knee straight and the thigh firm. The toes are soft and remain in contact with the floor. Keep your hips square or even to the front while pressing the knee open to

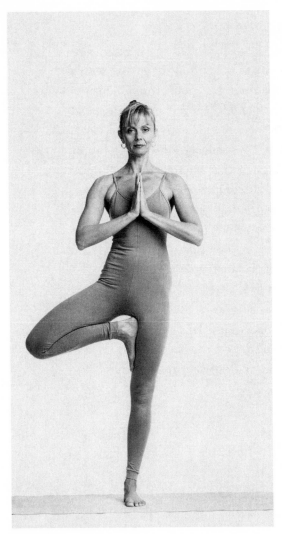

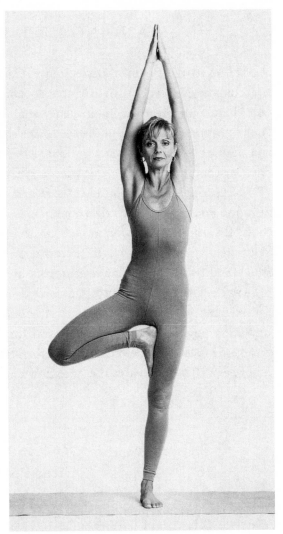

FIG. 78   FIG. 79

the side. Firm the buttocks and draw the abdominals in and up. Keep the chest lifted and the shoulders drawn down. Choose a spot in front of you and keep your attention focused on this spot. Hold for several breaths. When you are ready, release the leg and return to Tadasana. Pause here for a few breaths. Repeat on the other side.

REPETITIONS: Once or twice on both sides. Take your time. Moving in haste will likely defeat your balance.

MODIFICATIONS: If you can't seem to find your balance or the upper leg won't stay in place, lower the upper leg on the standing leg, or perform the pose at the wall. If you face the wall, lightly place the fingertips of both hands on the wall for support. If you stand with your side to the wall, the hand that touches the wall is on the same side as the standing or supporting leg.

IMAGE: From the waist down your body is like the roots of a tree, grounding into the Earth, and your upper torso—the branches and leaves of the tree—is lifting toward the sunshine.

EMPHASIS: On maintaining your equilibrium. Pay particular attention to your "focus"—both internal and external. The internal point of focus is the abdominal area, around the navel; the external point is the "spot" your eyes focus on.

BENEFITS: Develops balance, concentration, and hip-joint flexibility; promotes strength of character and willpower.

10

Seated Poses

The following sequence takes you back to the floor to balance the energizing effect of the standing poses and help prepare you for relaxation and meditation. The focus of this segment is on flexibility; however, we've also included a few poses to strengthen the arms. We recommend that you begin all seated poses by first coming into Sukhasana to adjust your hips and back and then moving into Dandasana to energize and place the legs properly.

SUKHASANA
Easy Seated Pose

ABOUT THE POSE: *Sukha* means joy, pleasure, or ease. As the name implies, this is the easiest of all the seated poses. Also known as Tailor's Pose, this posture introduces you to the technical aspects of the seated poses. Although the mechanics of this posture are quite simple, this pose may prove to be more challenging than it looks. The seated poses are often the most difficult for the adult beginner. Be patient. This posture enables you to discover tightness and weakness you didn't even know you had in your lower back, hips, and thighs.

LET'S PRACTICE

TECHNIQUE:

VARIATION 1: Sit on the floor and cross your legs, so that the feet are away from the buttocks and the lower legs are crossed between the ankles and the shins. (Figure 80.) If your knees seem to lift way up above the line of your pelvis and your lower back is rounding, or sinking, place a folded blanket or towel under you and sit at the front edge of it. As you become more flexible, you'll need less height, and you'll be able to reduce the thickness of the blanket or towel. Next, straighten your back, lifting up from the lower back, opening the chest, and pulling the shoulders back and down. Lengthen your neck and keep the chin parallel to the floor. Relax your hands on your thighs, palms face down. Remain here for a minute or two, focusing on your breathing. Then change and practice with the other leg crossed in front.

VARIATION 2: SEATED TWIST. Return to your first side. Place your left wrist or palm on your left knee and your right arm behind your right hip, palm flat on the floor. On the exhale, twist toward the right, looking over your right shoulder. (Figure 81.) Remain here for several breaths—lifting up through the crown of your head as you inhale, and increasing the twist as you exhale. Initiate the twist

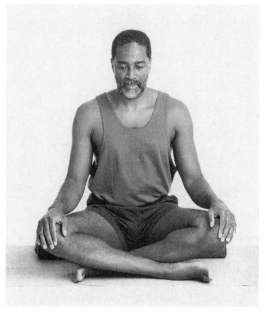

FIG. 80

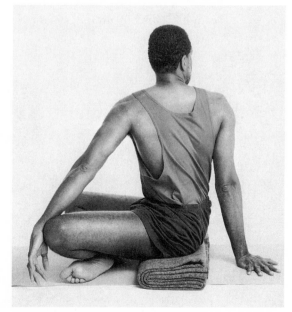

FIG. 81

from your waist, not your upper back. Slowly come out of the twist and cross your other leg in front, changing sides.

REPETITIONS: This posture may be practiced often and held for as long as is comfortable.

EMPHASIS: On lifting the chest and keeping the shoulders down. This facilitates the extension you want to achieve in all the seated postures.

BENEFITS: Strengthens muscles of the torso, both front and back; promotes flexibility in hip joints and lower back; and prepares you for all the seated poses as well as for meditation practice.

COUNTERPOSE: Apanasana, or Balasana (Child's Pose).

DANDASANA
Staff Pose

ABOUT THE POSE: *Danda* is a rod or staff. Although this posture may not look like much, it is one of the most dynamic of all the seated postures. As you sit on the floor with your legs straight in front of you, the spine is vertically aligned and at a right angle to the legs. As the name implies, the spine is "ram rod" straight. This posture is preparatory to all the seated forward bends.

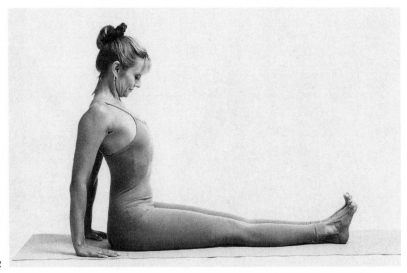

FIG. 82

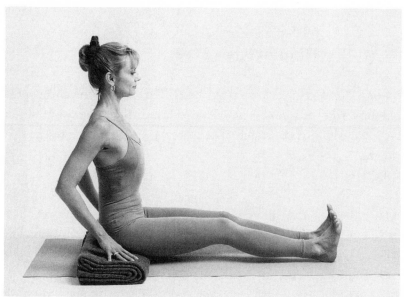

FIG. 83

LET'S PRACTICE

TECHNIQUE: Begin in Sukhasana (Easy Seated Pose). Keeping your back very straight, unfold your legs, stretching them straight out in front of you. Place your arms at your sides, hands flat on the floor, back a few inches from the line of your hips, and fingertips facing forward. Contract your thighs and lift your kneecaps. Flex your feet, drawing your toes back toward you and your heels away from you. Lift your chest and roll your shoulders back and down. Look down at your chest as you hold this pose. (Figure 82.) Breathe rhythmically.

REPETITIONS: Hold this posture for 5 to 10 breaths. Repeat between other seated postures.

MODIFICATIONS: If needed, sit on one or more folded blankets. It is more important to have the spine straight than the legs. So, if need be, bend the knees, keeping the feet flexed. (Figure 83.) Another option is to sit with your back to the wall.

EMPHASIS: On lifting the chest, engaging the back muscles, and extending from your sit bones to your heels through the backs of your legs.

BENEFITS: Strengthens the back, tones the arms, and stretches the hamstrings.

COUNTERPOSE: Forward bends such as Janusirsasana, or back-bending poses such as Chatushpada Pitham.

JANUSIRSASANA
Head-to-Knee Pose

ABOUT THE POSE: *Janu* is knee. *Sirsa* is the head. This pose is one of the most basic of the seated forward bends. *Janusirsasana* stretches the legs one at a time. In its classic form, it is a fairly intense stretch. Therefore we are going to present this posture in two stages.

LET'S PRACTICE

TECHNIQUE:

LEVEL 1: WITH PROPS. Sit on a folded blanket in Dandasana. Bend your left leg, bringing the sole of the foot as high up the inner right thigh as possible. The hips should remain in line with one another. Take your strap and place it over the bottom of the right foot. Take an end in each hand. The right foot is flexed with the knee straight. Keep the torso upright as you hold the strap and lift through the back. (Figure 84.) The shoulders are down, the chest is lifted, and the elbows are slightly bent. Hold here for several breaths. When you are ready, release the strap and change sides.

LEVEL 2: WITHOUT PROPS. Begin in Dandasana. Bend the left leg, bringing the heel toward the left sitting bone. Let the left leg drop to the side so it rests on the outer thigh and knee. Keep your right leg extended. Inhale and raise both arms overhead. Feel the lift originating from your sit bones. Exhale and bend forward from your hips, reaching the arms forward. Interlace the fingers and clasp the ball of the right foot. Keep the spine extended as you lower your chest toward your thigh and your face toward your knee. (Figure 85.) Hold for several breaths. When you are ready, release the hands, inhale, and come upright. Repeat to the other side.

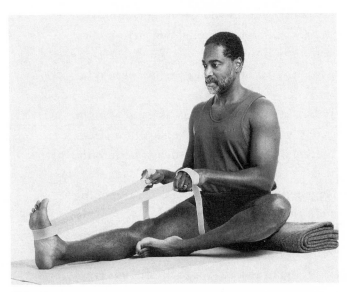

FIG. 84

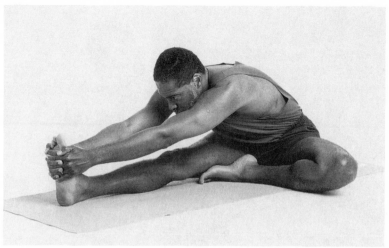

FIG. 85

REPETITIONS: Move slowly and hold each side for several breaths.

EMPHASIS: On lengthening the torso over the extended leg. Keep the opposite hip and thigh anchored as you move toward the extended leg.

BENEFITS: Stretches the extended leg, opens the hips, tones and stimulates the internal organs, strengthens and elongates the spine.

COUNTERPOSE: Either a backbend or a twist.

CONTRAINDICATIONS: Sciatica.

CHATUSHPADA PITHAM
Four-Legged Platform (Table Pose)

ABOUT THE POSE: *Chat* is the number four. *Pada* is foot. *Pitham* is platform. Often referred to as "Table Pose," this posture complements forward bends and, because it entails a degree of hyperextension, it will prepare you for back-bending poses. It resembles Two-Legged Platform Pose, which we learned earlier in our supine series, and, therefore, the mechanics of this pose are quite similar.

LET'S PRACTICE

TECHNIQUE: Beginning in Dandasana, bend your knees and place your feet hip-distance apart with toes pointing forward. Move your hands back about a hand space, approximately 6 to 8 inches, behind the line of your hips, separating them a little more than shoulder width. Keep the fingertips pointing forward. Inhale;

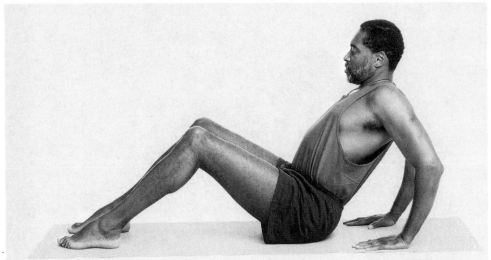

FIG. 86

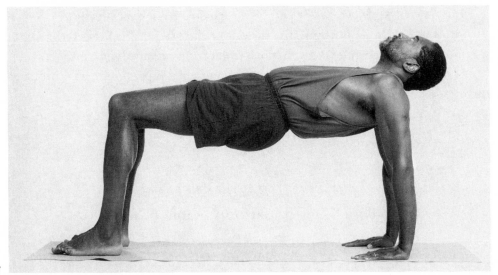

FIG. 87

bend your elbows slightly. (Figure 86.) As you exhale, peel your tailbone up from the floor just as you did in Dvipada Pitham, bringing the torso to a horizontal line, parallel to the floor. Let the head tilt back. (Figure 87.) If this is uncomfortable, keep the head up and look toward your knees. Straighten the arms and keep the wrists in line with the shoulders, the ankles in line with the knees. Contract your buttocks, maintaining a pelvic tilt. *Do not let the back or buttocks collapse or sag.* (Figure 88—incorrect.) Hold for 2 to 3 breaths. Lower down as you exhale.

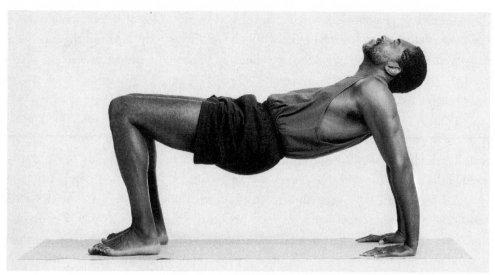

FIG. 88
(INCORRECT)

REPETITIONS: Repeat 2 or 3 times.

MODIFICATIONS: If your shoulder joints are particularly tight or your wrists are sensitive, vary the position of your hands. Either point your fingers out to the sides or to the back. You might even balance on your fists with the inner wrists facing one another.

EMPHASIS: On the back of the body—buttocks and hamstrings. Focus on lifting the pubic bone as high as possible.

BENEFITS: Tones and strengthens the arms and legs, stretches the muscles of the chest and·hip flexors.

COUNTERPOSE: Apanasana with both knees to chest.

CAUTIONS: If you are suffering from carpal tunnel syndrome, modify your hand position. If it places too much stress on your wrists, delete this practice from your repertoire.

PASCHIMOTTANASANA
Full Posterior Stretch (Seated Forward Bend)

ABOUT THE POSE: *Paschima* literally means "west." In yoga, the entire back, or posterior, of the body is considered the western part of the body. The front, or anterior, of the body is the east. The northern aspect is given to the top, or crown, of the head; while the southern aspect is applied to the soles of the feet. *Paschimottanasana* is an intense stretch of the whole back of the body. Because this can be a very challenging stretch, we offer two stages of progression for its practice.

LET'S PRACTICE

TECHNIQUE:

LEVEL 1: Follow the directions for Dandasana, sitting on a folded blanket. Also use a strap, placing it over the bottoms of your feet and holding an end in each hand. Hold this position for several breaths. When you are ready to bend forward, inhale and lift through the crown of the head. Exhale and begin to draw your torso forward over your thighs, leading with your chest. Your elbows will bend relative to the degree that you are bringing your torso forward. Keep your shoulders relaxed, your knees straight, and the feet flexed. Remember to bend from your hips, not the waist. (Figure 89.) Contract the quadriceps and maintain as much extension as possible from your tailbone to the top of your head. Hold here for several breaths. When you are ready to come out, inhale and lift upright. Exhale and release the strap.

LEVEL 2: THE CLASSIC POSE. You are ready for this version when, from Dandasana, you can hold onto your feet with your hands while keeping both your legs and your back straight. From Dandasana, inhale and lift your arms out and up overhead. Interlace your fingers and turn your palms toward the ceiling. Pause

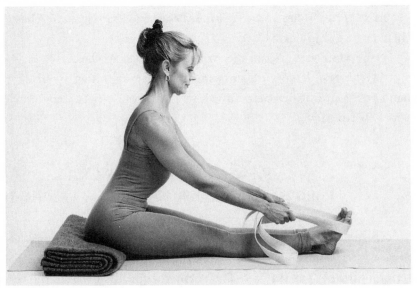

FIG. 89

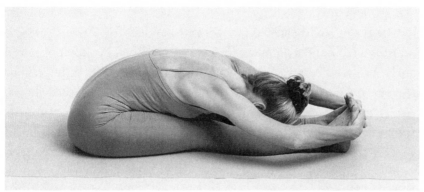

FIG. 90

here and exhale. Inhale, stretch up once again. As you exhale extend your arms down toward your feet. Clasp the hands over the balls of the feet, interlocking the fingers, and extend the torso over the thighs so that the forehead rests on the shins. (Figure 90.) Hold for several breaths. To come up, release your hands, inhale, and come upright. Exhale and relax here for a few breaths.

REPETITIONS: Approach this posture slowly. Take several breaths at each stage of its progression. Ultimately this pose is held for 1 to 5 minutes. Practice once or twice within a sequence, performing a counterpose in between your efforts.

EMPHASIS: On keeping the spine extended or straight and bending from the hips. Focus on reaching the chest up and over the thighs.

BENEFITS: Increases flexibility in the entire posterior musculature, stretches the hamstrings and back muscles, massages the abdominal organs, and has a calming effect on the whole body and mind.

COUNTERPOSE: The following posture, *Purvottanasana,* is the perfect mate to this pose.

CONTRAINDICATIONS: Sciatica.

PURVOTTANASANA
Full Anterior Stretch

ABOUT THE POSE: *Purvo* means "east." *Uttana* is intense. This posture stretches the eastern, or front, part of the body, making it a perfect counterpose to Paschimottanasana, which stretches the western, or back, part of the body.

LET'S PRACTICE

TECHNIQUE: Begin in Dandasana and place your hands 8 to 10 inches behind the line of your hips with fingers pointing forward. Inhale, bend your elbows, and lean back slightly into your hands. (Figure 91.) As you exhale, press through your heels and lift your buttocks off the floor, straightening through the elbows. While the torso is in a horizontal position, parallel to the floor, the legs form a slanted line from the tops of the thighs down to the toes. The ankles and knees stay together. The toes point to reach the floor. Contract your buttocks and thighs and keep your kneecaps facing up. Press down through the arms into the hands as well as into the heels. Lift through the pubic bone and sternum and release the head back, if it's comfortable. (Figure 92.) Hold for several breaths, breathing rhythmically. *Take care not to collapse in the chest or pelvis.* (Figure 93— incorrect.) When you are ready to come down, exhale and release the buttocks to the floor.

REPETITIONS: Repeat 2 or 3 more times.

MODIFICATIONS: If the shoulders are tight and the wrists are weak, vary the position of the hands like you did in Chatushpada Pitham or use your fists. Practicing this pose with the balls of the feet on the wall will help properly activate the legs.

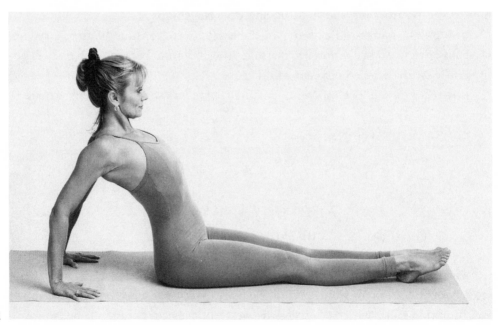

FIG. 91

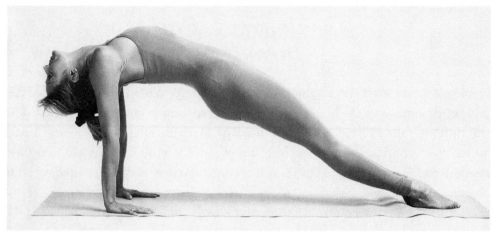

FIG. 92

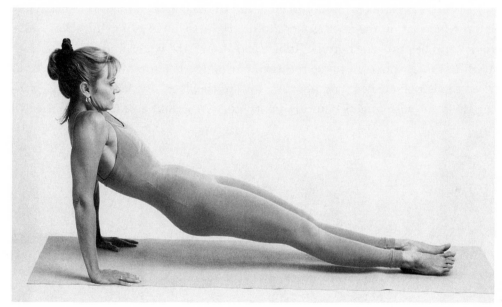

FIG. 93
(INCORRECT)

EMPHASIS: On the lift of the pubic bone and the chest. To keep your legs from rolling out, imagine that your ankles and knees are tied together.

BENEFITS: Strengthens the wrists, ankles, and posterior musculature; enhances flexibility in the shoulder joints; expands chest.

COUNTERPOSE: Paschimottanasana or any other forward-bending posture.

MARICHYASANA III
Seated Twist

ABOUT THE POSE: A mythical character, the sage Marichi was the son of the creator, Brahma, and the grandfather of Surya (the sun god). This seated twist is the third of four twisted poses dedicated to Marichi. One of the many seated twists, this variation involves the bending of one leg while keeping the other leg straight out in front of you. In its full form, this twist is quite challenging for beginners, so we offer two simpler variations.

LET'S PRACTICE

TECHNIQUE:

LEVEL 1: Sitting on a folded blanket in Dandasana, bend the right knee, placing the foot flat on the floor as close to the right sit bone as possible. Place your right hand behind your buttock. Inhale and stretch the left arm up to the ceiling. With an exhalation, turn to the right, and bring the left arm over the right thigh. Keep the left elbow bent and pointing toward the floor. The left palm is flat, facing the right with fingers pointing up. (Figure 94.) Hold here for a few breaths.

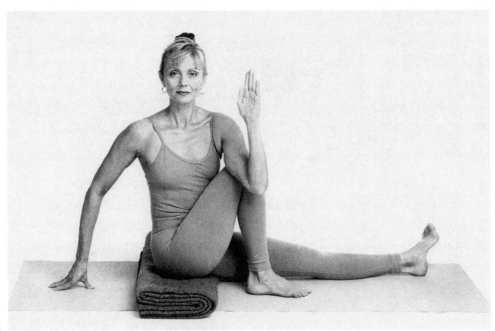

FIG. 94

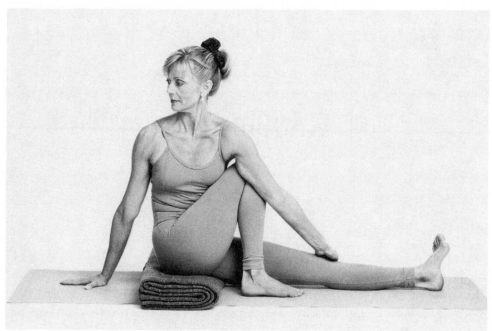

FIG. 95

LEVEL 2: Take hold of the outer side of the left shin with the left hand. Look over your right shoulder. (Figure 95.) Hold here for several breaths.

REPETITIONS: One set of this pose is sufficient.

EMPHASIS: On extending up through the spine on the inhalation and increasing the twist on the exhalation. On twisting from the navel, not the upper back or neck.

BENEFITS: Serves as an antidote to lower back and hip joint discomfort, encourages shoulder joint flexibility and mobility in the neck or cervical vertebrae, massages the abdominal area, and enhances the functioning of the internal organs. It tones the waist and, with regular practice, reduces both the sluggishness in, and the size of, the abdomen.

11

Abdominals

A strong abdominal musculature is indispensable to good posture, coordination, and balance. Consciously engaging your abdominals both supports and protects your back, keeping you free from injury, while reducing the chronic back pain associated with a sedentary lifestyle. Although it may seem that the repertoire of hatha yoga doesn't include poses specifically to strengthen the abdominal musculature, there are actually several yoga postures that engage this portion of the anatomy.

The abdominal musculature has four components. The rectus abdominis attaches to the pubic bone and runs up the center of the torso, connecting to the sternum and lower ribs at the top. It controls forward flexion of the torso. You engage this muscle, for instance, in the Cat Stretch when you round your back, drawing your head toward your pubic bone. The transverse abdominals wrap around the spine horizontally, like a cummerbund. This muscle is activated when you emphasize the exhalation, drawing the navel toward the backbone, as you do in the Breath of Fire breathing exercise. The other two components of the abdominals are the internal and external obliques, which crisscross at each side of your waist. You engage these muscles each time you perform a spinal twist and they assist in lateral flexion when you bend to the side. The following posture dramatically exercises the obliques, as well as the transverse abdominals.

JATHARA PARIVARTANASANA
Twisted Stomach Pose

ABOUT THE POSE: *Jathara* means stomach or belly. *Parivartana* means turning or rolling about. A supine posture, this pose engages the transverse and oblique abdominal musculature, as well as the inner and outer thighs (adductors and abductors) and the hamstrings. Torsion takes place in the spine as the legs are lowered and lifted to each side of you. Each increment of the following series adds another degree of challenge. Stage 4 demonstrates the classical variation.

LET'S PRACTICE

TECHNIQUE:

Stage 1: Begin in Basic Supine position, with your knees and ankles together and your feet flat on the floor. Bend your elbows and clasp your hands underneath your head, palms cupping the base of your skull. Inhale. Feel as though your ankles and knees are tied together, throughout this exercise. On an exhale, draw your knees over to the right and look straight ahead or to your left. The outside edge of the right foot will remain in contact with the floor. At no time, in this

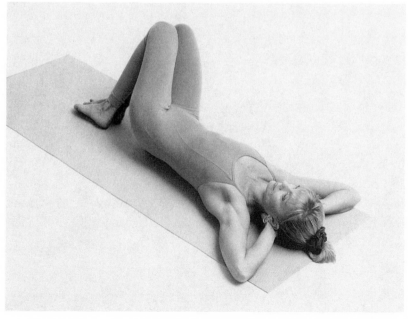

FIG. 96

variation, are both feet fully lifted from the floor. Your knees will move about halfway or less to the side. (Figure 96.) Do not press your knees all the way to the floor. Hold here and inhale. Exhale as you return your knees and head center. Pause center, inhale. Continue on, repeating the directions to the left.

Stage 2: Bring your arms to a "T-square," shoulder level on the floor, palms facing down. On an exhale, bring your legs up, keeping the knees bent. (Figure 97.) Your knees will be above your hips and your shins slightly higher than parallel to the floor. The feet are passive and the head remains center. Inhale and, with knees together, move the legs about halfway, or less, to the right. (Figure 98.) The left buttock will lift up slightly. Keep the left shoulder down. Exhale, bring the knees center. Repeat to the left side.

Stage 3: Begin with your knees bent. Inhale and bring your knees to the right, as you did in Stage 2. Keeping your thighs and knees absolutely stationary, exhale and straighten your lower legs from this angle. (Figure 99.) Keep the

FIG. 97

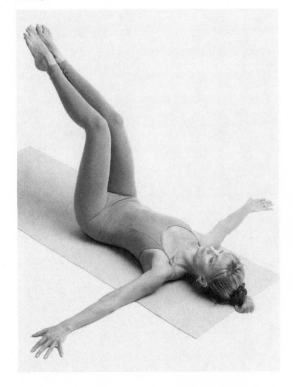

FIG. 98

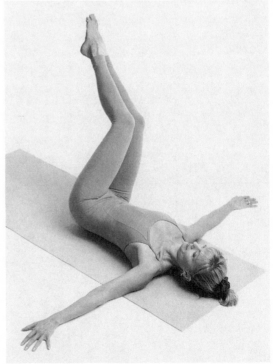

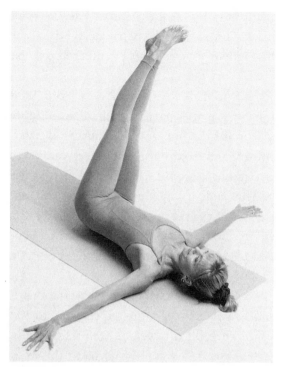

FIG. 99

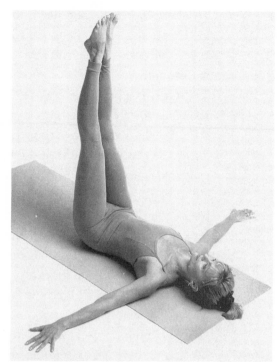

FIG. 100

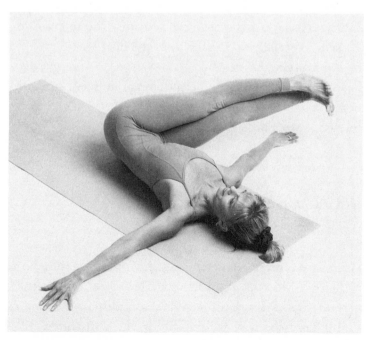

FIG. 101

left shoulder down. The left buttock will only lift slightly. Inhale and, keeping the legs at this angle, bend your lower legs. Engage the hamstrings and draw the lower buttocks together as you do this. Exhale as you return center. Repeat on the left side.

Stage 4: The Classic Pose. Begin as you have for stages 2 & 3. Straighten your legs toward the ceiling above your hips, perpendicular to the floor. (Figure 100.) Inhale. Exhale, lowering the legs toward the fingertips of your right hand. As you do this keep your head center or turn and look to the left. Keep your knees and ankles together and your knees straight. (Figure 101.) Hold here for a few breaths. Continue to energize the legs and, if you can, keep the feet from resting on the floor. At the same time turn your navel or stomach in the opposite direction to the feet. Your left shoulder stays on the floor. Exhale as you bring your legs back to center. Take a full breath in place and then proceed to the left.

REPETITIONS: Practice each stage 2 or 3 times.

MODIFICATIONS: Keeping your knees together in all of these variations is very important. This helps you to strengthen your inner thighs. If the structure of your legs prevents you from doing this, place a rolled towel, or even a small rubber ball, in between your knees or thighs. If you feel stress in your back, this exercise may simply be too difficult for you at this time. Stay with the stages you can perform well. In stages 2 and 3 you may want to bring the knees a little closer to the body to accommodate your back. At the beginning, in the Classic Pose, you may want to bend your knees, especially on the lift from the floor.

PREPARATION FOR: All twisting poses.

BENEFITS: Strengthens transverse and oblique abdominal muscles, strengthens adductors and abductors.

COUNTERPOSE: Apanasana with both knees to chest.

PARIPURNA NAVASANA
Full Boat Pose

ABOUT THE POSE: *Paripurna* means whole or complete. *Nava* is a ship, boat, or vessel. Balancing on the buttocks, this posture resembles a boat with oars. A challenging pose in its full form, this posture requires a certain amount of strength in the back and hip flexors as well as flexibility in the hamstrings.

LET'S PRACTICE

TECHNIQUE:

Stage 1: Sit on the floor or your mat with your knees bent and your feet flat on the floor in front of you, hip-distance apart. Place your fingertips underneath your knees from the outside. Inhale the breath as you draw yourself forward onto your sit bones, lifting the chest and into the crown of the head. (Figure 102.) Shoulders are down, and chin is level to the floor. As you exhale, draw backward, rounding your back as you move toward the back of your buttocks. You are in a rounded, Cat Back, position. Keep your shoulders down. Look toward your navel. (Figure 103.) Hold here for a few breaths. Keep your thighs as relaxed as possible. When you are ready, return to center on an inhalation.

Stage 2: The Classic Pose. Repeat Stage 1. Hold on to your knees for a breath or two. On an exhalation, straighten your legs from the knees and extend your arms forward. (Figure 104.) Hold

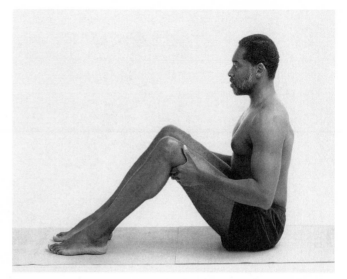

FIG. 102

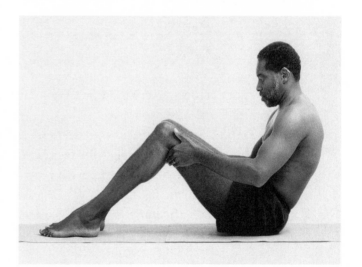

FIG. 103

and breathe. Your legs are now close together, and the arms are parallel to the floor. Keep the shoulders down and the arms taut. Now lift your chin, slightly, and look toward your big toes. Your feet will be higher than the level of your head. Keep your chest lifted and your back as straight as possible. To complete, bring your fingertips under your knees, draw your legs to your chest, and place the feet on the floor.

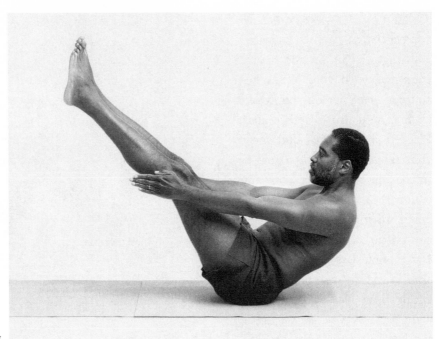

FIG. 104

REPETITIONS: Repeat Stage 1 two to five times before proceeding to Stage 2. Practice Stage 2 once or twice.

BENEFITS: Strengthens the transverse and rectus abdominis muscles, hip flexors, and the lower back; tones the legs; and promotes relief of gastric complaints.

COUNTERPOSE: Apanasana with both knees to chest, Chatushpada Pitham, and Purvottanasana.

CAUTIONS: If Stage 2 puts too much of a strain on your back, just do Stage 1.

12

Inversions

Inverting the body is an important aspect of yoga asana. The ultimate inversion, of course, is Headstand. But there are many ways to invert the body, and you've already experienced three poses that do that to some degree: Uttanasana (Standing Forward Bend), Prasarita Padottanasana (Spread Legs Intense Forward Bend), and Downward-Facing Dog. Although these are not full-body inversions, they provide you with some of the same benefits: reversing the effects of gravity, relieving the pressure on the abdominal organs, and enhancing circulation to the upper chest and head. Practice of Headstand, Shoulderstand, and Plough provides additional benefits to the glandular system, but these poses are best learned from a competent teacher. Improperly learned, they can lead to neck and back strain. *Viparita Karani Mudra,* will give you a taste of what an inversion feels like.

VIPARITA KARANI MUDRA
Inverted Pose

Viparita Karani literally means "in the inverted manner." While it looks a lot like Shoulderstand, it's different in a couple of important ways: The neck bears less weight, and the back muscles are less active. The hands support the lower back behind the waist, directing circulation to this area before it travels down to the chest and head. Many people prefer practicing this pose at the wall.

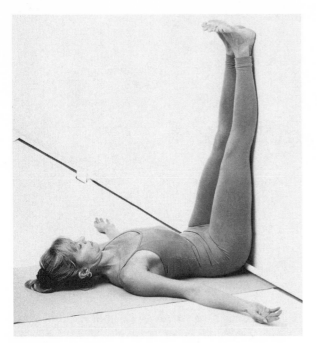

FIG. 105

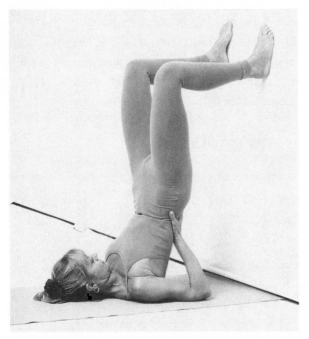

FIG. 106

LET'S PRACTICE

TECHNIQUE:

Stage 1: Sit on the floor with one side close to the wall. Using your hands and arms to support you, reach your legs up the wall and lower your back to the floor. Square your sit bones to the wall and position your buttocks approximately 6 inches from the baseboard (less if you're more flexible). Extend your legs up the wall and either straighten your knees or keep them bent. (Figure 105.) Breathe abdominally for several breaths.

Stage 2: Bend your knees so that your feet are flat against the wall, hip-distance apart. Place your arms next to your hips, palms flat on the floor. On an exhale, slowly peel the spine off the floor, using the strength in the backs of your legs. Press into your heels and the balls of your feet and keep your toes soft. Hold this position with thighs aligned vertically and shins parallel to the floor, for 2 to 3 breaths, and gently lower down as you exhale.

Stage 3: Repeat Stage 2, but with the following variation: Place your hands behind your waist, with the palms flat against your body and your fingers spread, and bring your elbows toward one another behind your back. (Figure 106.) On an exhale, raise one leg from the wall. (Figure 107.) Stay for a couple of breaths. Return the leg to the wall and extend the other leg.

When you feel secure, raise both legs from the wall. The legs are straight and slightly forward from your hips, with your toes above your forehead. Look toward your feet and breathe. To come out of the pose, reverse the movements.

Stage 4: The Classic Pose: Done in the center of the room, this pose is quite similar to Stage 3. Begin in Basic Supine and bring your knees up to your chest. Roll the hips off the floor and place your hands behind your waist with your elbows moving toward one another. Slowly straighten your legs and direct the toes above the line of your face. (Figure 108.) Hold for several breaths and slowly reverse the movement to come out of the pose.

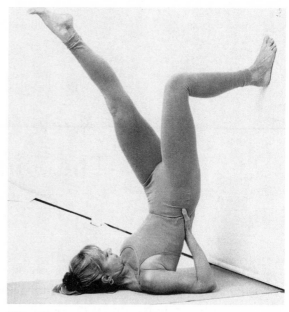

FIG. 107

REPETITIONS: Practice Stage 1 once and hold it for at least 30 to 60 seconds; Stage 2 three to five times; and Stages 3 and 4 once or twice. Once you become comfortable in the pose, just practice Stage 4.

PREPARATION FOR: More advanced inversions such as Shoulderstand.

BENEFITS: Enhances circulation and functioning of female organs; relieves congestion in the legs; and is an excellent antidote for lower back discomfort.

CONTRAINDICATIONS: Do not practice this posture during menstruation or pregnancy, if you suffer from high or low blood pressure, glaucoma, or detached retina, or if you have congestion in the ears.

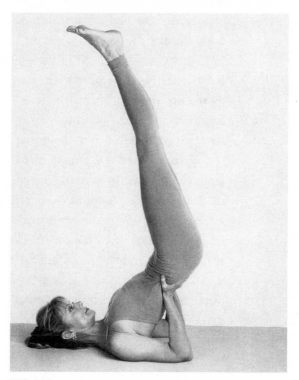

FIG. 108

13

Surya Namaskar—
The Sun Salutation

Apparently a more recent tradition in the realm of classical hatha yoga, the Sun Salute, or Salutation to the Sun, a series of 12 postures performed in sequence, is believed to have been developed and incorporated into the repertoire within the last 100 years. As the name implies, this series is done in the morning as a kind of prayer of the body, expressing reverence for life while accessing the power and energy of the sun.

The poses of Sun Salute are performed according to the principle of pose and counterpose. Because there is a continual flow of movement, Sun Salute also represents the dynamic principle in the approach to asana. Made up of both forward- and back-bending poses, this sequence creates a perfect balance of strength and flexibility to the musculature of the whole front and back of the body.

With the added element of continual movement for a specified number of repetitions, you also have the component of stamina. Practiced regularly, this classic series has the potential to contribute significantly to cardiovascular fitness.

Although not a full body workout by any means, Sun Salute has become an important element in the repertoire of most hatha yogis. At the same time, note that the form and details of Sun Salute vary according to the different systems that use it. The Sun Salute of the Ashtanga style, the most dramatically different from the classical variation, involves transitions that include jumps, which make this version even more dynamic. Because the Sun Salute may be overwhelming to the adult beginner, we have presented it here in two stages: modified and classical.

Let's practice!

MODIFIED SUN SALUTE

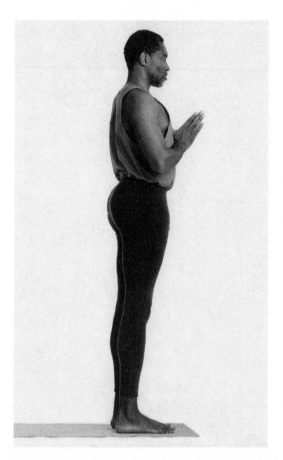

FIGURE 109–BASIC STANCE (TADASANA)
Stand in Basic Stance, feet hip-distance apart and hands in prayer position at your heart center. Inhale as you open your arms to the sides at shoulder level.

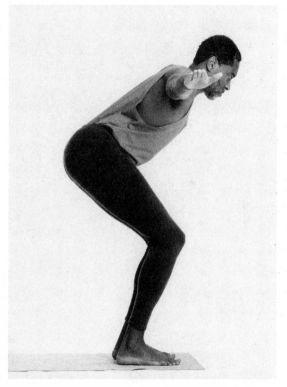

FIGURE 110–MODIFIED FORWARD BEND
Exhale, bend your knees, and bring your torso forward about 30 degrees. Pause here and inhale.

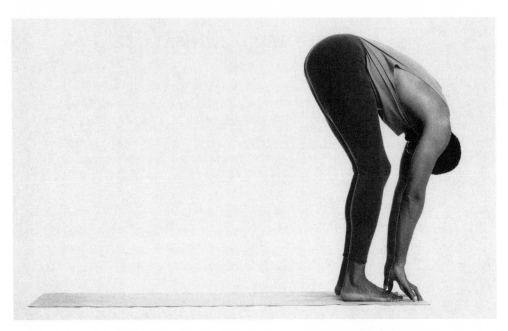

FIGURE 111–FORWARD BEND (UTTANASANA) Exhale and release your torso and arms down over your legs. Keep your knees bent, head down, and neck relaxed.

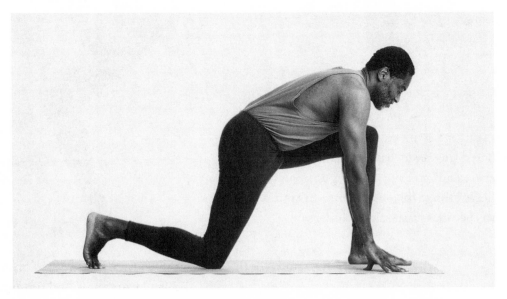

FIGURE 112–LUNGE Inhale, stretch your right leg back, place the knee down, and rest on the ball of your foot. Keep head lifted.

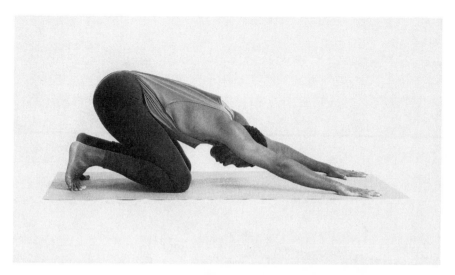

FIGURE 113–HALF-TORTOISE (BALASANA) Bring your left leg back in line with your right. Pressing into the balls of the feet, exhale as you pull back toward your heels. Keep your arms outstretched and lower your head.

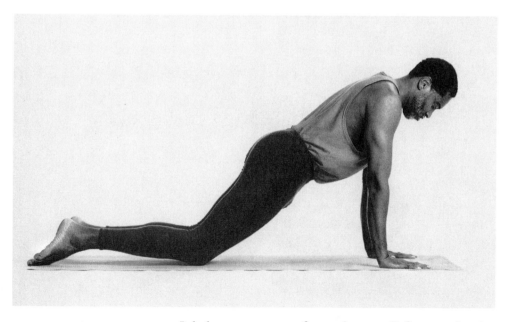

FIGURE 114–HALF PLANK Inhale as you come forward onto all fours and point your toes. Exhale, shifting your hips forward and down until your spine forms a slanted line. Draw the abdominals in and up. Hold here and inhale.

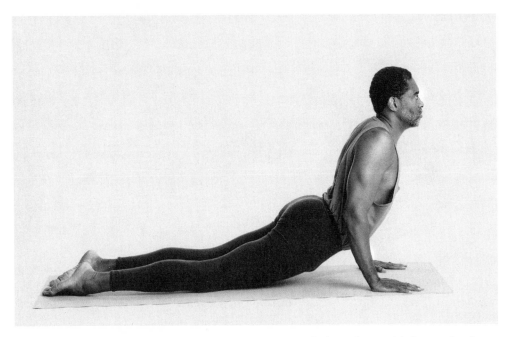

FIGURE 115–COBRA (BHUJANGASANA) On an exhale, release thighs to the floor. Lift chest and bend elbows slightly. Hold here and inhale.

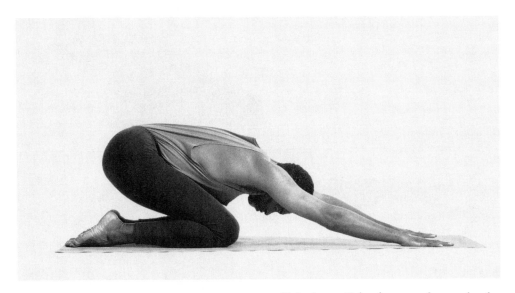

FIGURE 116–HALF-TORTOISE (BALASANA) Exhale; pull back toward your heels, pointing your toes. Inhale and return to all fours.

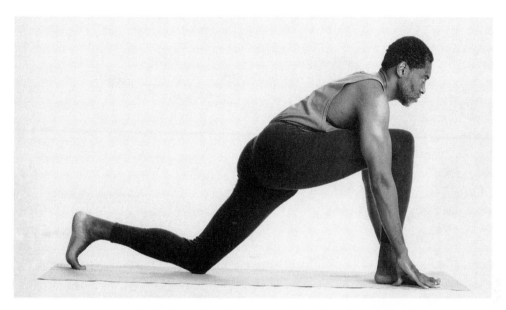

FIGURE 117–LUNGE Exhale, and bring your right foot forward in between your hands. Inhale.

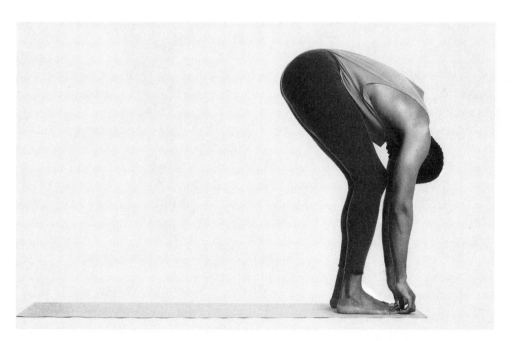

FIGURE 118–FORWARD BEND (UTTANASANA) Tuck your left foot under and, on an exhale, bring it forward to meet the right. Keep your head relaxed and knees bent.

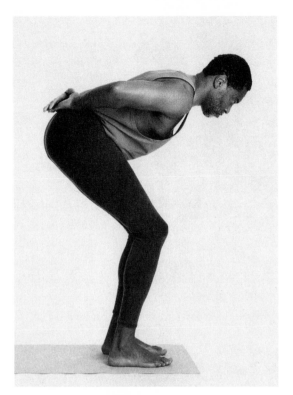

**FIGURE 119–RETURNING TO BASIC STANCE
(TADASANA)** With your knees bent, lift up
through the crown of your head, on an
inhalation, to a flat back. Place your hands on
your lower back as you come up. Exhale.

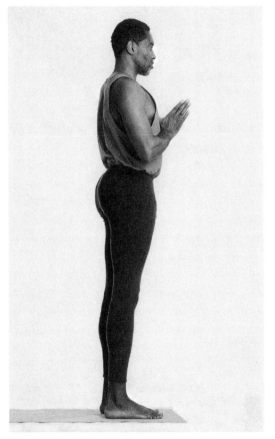

FIGURE 120–BASIC STANCE (TADASANA)
Inhale and return to Tadasana with hands in
prayer position. Exhale. Repeat entire
sequence with left leg initiating the lunge
back and the return forward.

CLASSIC SUN SALUTE

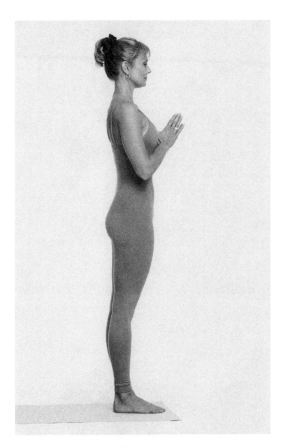

FIGURE 121–BASIC STANCE (TADASANA) Begin with hands at your heart in prayer position.

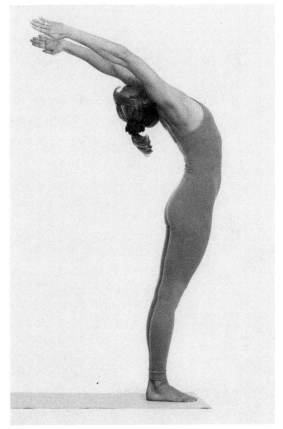

FIGURE 122–BACKBEND Inhale as you stretch your arms up as you arch back, keeping your legs and buttocks firm.

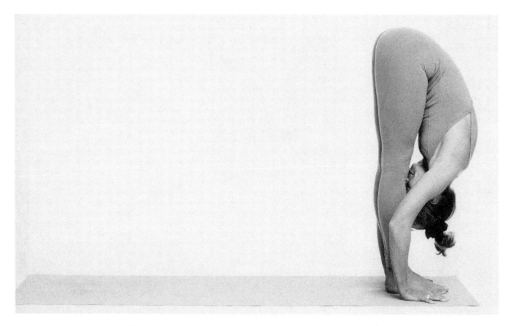

FIGURE 123–FORWARD BEND (UTTANASANA) Exhaling, stretch forward and down. Place hands outside your feet, with palms flat and fingers in line with toes. Draw your head in toward your knees.

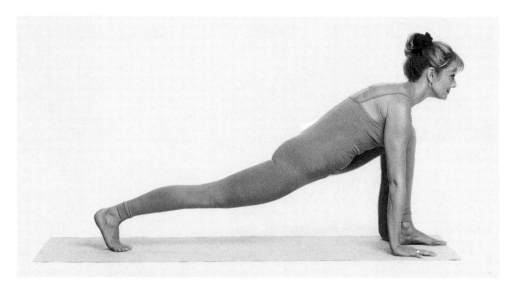

FIGURE 124–LUNGE Inhale and reach your right leg straight back to the ball of the foot. Lift your head and chest. Hold the breath in.

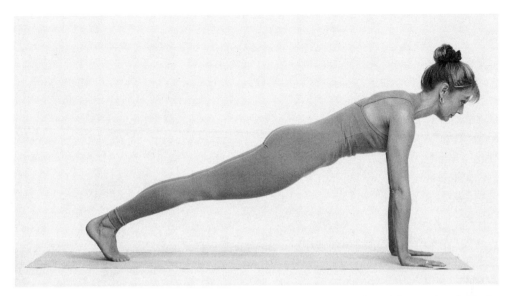

FIGURE 125–PLANK (CHATURANGA DANDASANA) Still holding the breath, reach your left leg back to meet the right. Legs should be straight and abdominals firm. Look down at the floor.

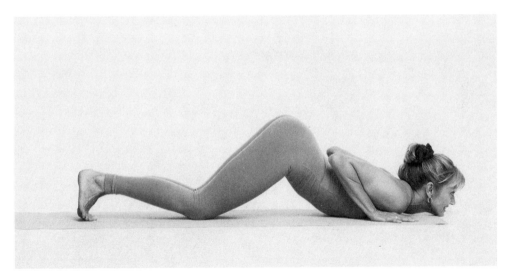

FIGURE 126–POSE OF EIGHT POINTS Exhaling, bend your elbows and lower your knees, chest, and chin to the floor. Arch your back and lift your buttocks. This transitional move may feel awkward at first. With practice it should flow into the next pose, Cobra.

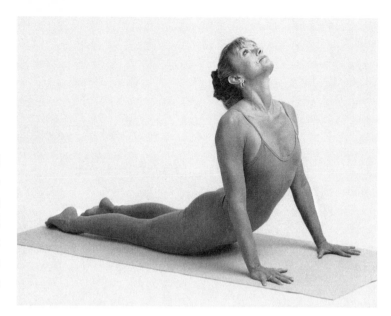

FIGURE 127–COBRA POSE (BHUJANGASANA)
Lower your hips, inhale, and lift your chest. Keep your elbows bent and pressed into your ribs. Hips, legs, and feet stay on the floor. Look up. Press shoulders down away from earlobes and firm the buttocks.

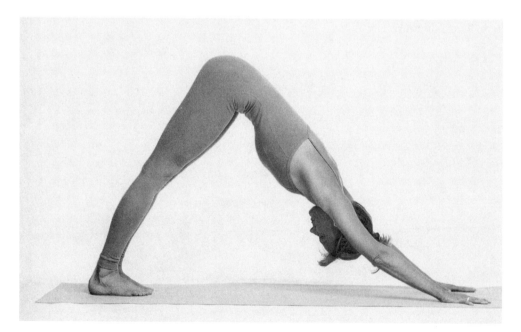

FIGURE 128–DOWNWARD-FACING DOG (ADHO MUKHA SVANASANA) Tuck your toes under and, on the exhale, press up and back to an inverted V position. Neck is relaxed in between the arms. Lengthen spine, firm thighs, straighten knees, and press heels down.

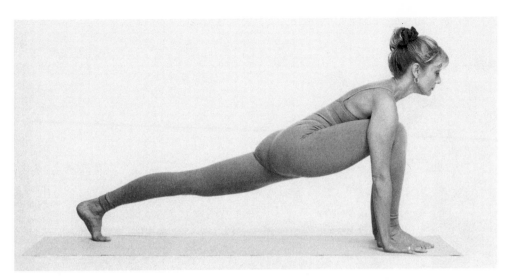

FIGURE 129–LUNGE Lift your head and, inhaling, bring your right foot forward in between your hands.

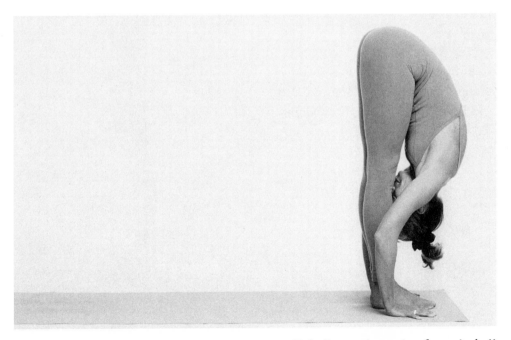

FIGURE 130–FORWARD BEND (UTTANASANA) Exhaling and pressing from the ball of the left foot, bring your left leg forward to meet your right. Straighten your knees and place your hands, palms flat, on the outside of your feet.

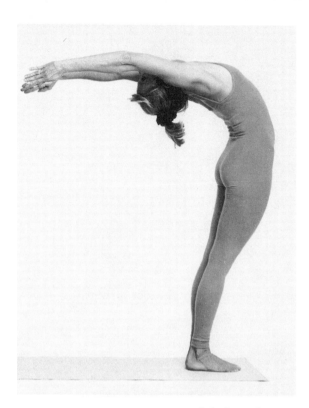

FIGURE 131–ARCHING BACK Inhale and come up with a straight back, arms alongside the head and neck. Knees remain straight, abdominals lifted. Look up and arch back.

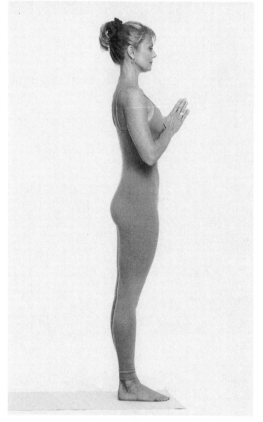

FIGURE 132–BASIC STANCE (TADASANA) Exhale as you return to Tadasana, hands at your heart. Repeat entire sequence with left leg initiating the lunge back and the return forward.

14

Relaxation

Traditionally, a period of relaxation completes a yoga session. The posture is called Corpse Pose and may be thought of as a counterpose to the class as a whole. Consider it your dessert!

This state of deep relaxation quiets the mind and allows the body to rest in a reclining position on the floor. The eyes are closed and the breathing is natural. The mind remains observant and free from any concerns. You simply "watch" yourself while allowing your body to completely relax.

This deep level of rest is accompanied by a keen awareness of the process. Although it is not meant to replace sleep, afterward you will feel refreshed and energized.

SAVASANA
Corpse Pose

ABOUT THE POSE: *Sava* is a corpse. Dead Man's Pose, or the classic relaxation posture, traditionally completes all hatha yoga sessions. Lying supine on the floor, the body is symmetrically aligned, yet at rest. Although this posture may appear to be easy, it is actually one of the most challenging of all the poses to truly master.

LET'S PRACTICE

POSITION: Lie on your back, legs outstretched, in a comfortable and symmetrical way. As with your other supine postures, use a folded towel under the head to extend the neck, if necessary. Your chin points slightly downward, and the throat is soft. Close your eyes and draw your shoulders down from the earlobes. Place your arms at your sides with palms facing up to gently open the chest. Legs are slightly apart with the feet naturally falling open to each side. (Figure 133.) Once you are satisfied with your placement, remain here without disturbing your body for the duration of your relaxation.

TECHNIQUE: Begin by generally noting how you feel. Scan your body from the top of your head down to your feet. Take note of your breathing, the quality of your energy, and the existence of any stress, tension, or fatigue. Take a few deep, conscious, abdominal breaths at this point. As you exhale, allow any residual effort to leave your body and mind. Return to normal breathing. Again take a few deeper, abdominal breaths and with each exhalation let go of any unwanted tension and fatigue. Return to normal, silent breathing. Remain here for several minutes. Continue to observe yourself, breathing naturally. If you find your mind wandering or getting caught up in thought, simply take some deeper breaths and consciously let go of any and all physical effort or mental agitation.

Always come out of your relaxation slowly. Begin by moving your fingers and toes and bringing your awareness back to the room. When you are ready, bend your knees and slowly roll to your side. Pause here for a breath or two. Bring yourself to a seated position. Sit for a minute or two before you stand up.

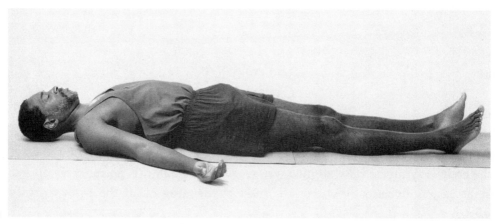

FIG. 133

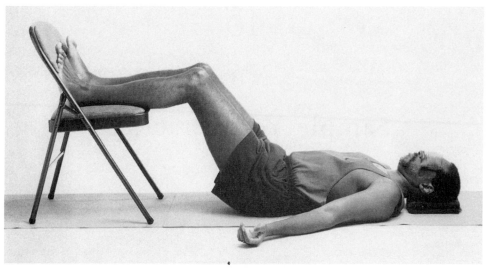

FIG. 134

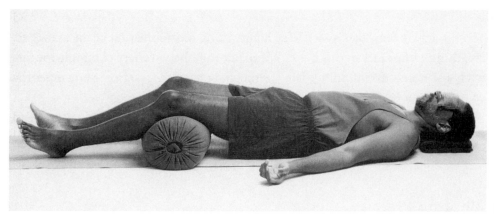

FIG. 135

REPETITIONS: Make Savasana the last part of your practice, allowing anywhere from 5 minutes to 20 minutes. Practice Savasana anytime you feel stress,
undue fatigue, or want to take a break from your daily routine.

MODIFICATIONS: Note that you do not have to have your back flat or pressed
to the floor. However, if you tend to have an exaggerated lumbar curve (i.e., sway
back, when standing), you may then want to add a rolled towel or blanket underneath your knees, or prop your feet up on a padded chair. (Figure 134.) This will
allow your back to soften naturally into the floor. For a supported Savasana, place
a bolster under your knees, a folded towel under your head, and an eyebag over
your eyes. (Figure 135.)

15

Sample Yoga Practices

You can create your own practice at home, using a combination of the asanas and breathing techniques in this book. We've put together a variety of sample routines to choose from—for morning, late afternoon, or evening practice. Remember that you can add a period of meditation to any of them. Enjoy!

Greeting the Day

Morning Practice

A morning routine should begin gently with some back stretches and slowly accelerate to a more energizing sequence. It works best if you take a hot shower or warm bath before starting your practice, or even begin with a brisk 15-minute walk to warm you up.

Practice the following asanas in dynamic fashion, using the breath to move into, and out of, each pose several times.

Prone Poses

CHAKRAVAKASANA (CAT STRETCH) Inhale as you arch; exhale on the contraction. See Figures 37 and 38, pages 83 and 84.

BALASANA (CHILD'S POSE; HALF-TORTOISE VARIATION) Exhale as you move back into pose. See Figure 40, pages 84 and 85.

BHUJANGASANA (COBRA) Inhale as you come to all fours; exhale down to floor; inhale to come into pose; exhale and return to Half-Tortoise. See Figure 47, pages 88 and 89.

Standing Poses

SURYA NAMASKAR (MODIFIED OR CLASSIC SUN SALUTATION) Do one to three sets of either version, or a combination of both. Remember that one set means doing the pose twice—once on each side. The first side begins with the right leg lunging back and finishes with the right leg coming forward; the second begins and ends with the left leg initiating the movement. Stand in Tadasana (Basic Stance) for at least a minute to complete the series. See Figures 109–32, pages 143–54.

SAVASANA (CORPSE POSE) Relax completely; or skip this pose and continue on. See Figures 133–35, pages 155–57.

Optional Sequence

TADASANA (BASIC STANCE) Take a few deep abdominal breaths. See Figures 52 and 53, pages 93 and 94.

UTKATASANA (CHAIR POSE) Either Bikram Choudhury's variation or B. K. S. Iyengar's. Come out of the pose on an inhalation. See Figures 57 and 58, pages 97–99.

UTTANASANA (FORWARD BEND) Initiate the forward bend on an exhalation. See Figures 60 and 61, pages 99–101.

TRIKONASANA (TRIANGLE POSE) Step or jump the feet to the proper stance (Figures 65A and B–67, pages 103 and 104); inhale, lift the arms to sides; exhale, move out and down; inhale to come up. See Figures 68–71, pages 105–8.

UTTANASANA (FORWARD BEND) Step or jump feet together; exhale forward. See Figures 60 and 61, pages 99–101.

PARSVAKONASANA (EXTENDED SIDE ANGLE STRETCH) Step or jump to wide stance. Inhale, lift arms to sides; exhale, moving out and down; breathe naturally; inhale to come up. See Figures 74 and 75, pages 110–12.

UTTANASANA (FORWARD BEND) Step or jump feet together; exhale forward. See Figures 60 and 61, pages 99–101.

VRKSASANA (TREE POSE) Inhale, bring heel to thigh; exhale, place hands at heart; breathe deeply for several breaths. See Figures 78 and 79, pages 115–17.

SAVASANA (CORPSE POSE) Relax completely. See Figures 133–35, pages 155–57.

Pause and Refresh

Midday or Late Afternoon Practice

Although this set of postures can be done anytime, it's particularly relaxing and refreshing after a long day. Spend a minute or more in each pose.

At the Wall

DOWNWARD-FACING DOG PREPARATION With hands pressing against wall. See Figure 49, pages 90–92.

UTKATASANA (CHAIR POSE) With back against the wall. See Figure 59, pages 97–99.

DANDASANA (STAFF POSE) With back against the wall. Figures 82 and 83, pages 120 and 121.

VIPARITA KARANI MUDRA (INVERTED POSE) Do entire progression at the wall and final pose away from wall. [Caution: If menstruating, do Stage 1 of this progression with only your legs extended up the wall.] See Figures 105–7, pages 139–41.

NOTE: If you would like to continue on, add the following poses to your sequence:

Standing Poses

CHOUDHURY'S ARDHA CHANDRASANA (HALF-MOON) Both right and left sides. See Figures 54 and 55, pages 95–97.

UTTANASANA (FORWARD BEND) Breathe deeply and stay in the pose for several breaths. See Figures 60 and 61, pages 99–101.

HINDI SQUAT Either modified with props or the full pose. See Figures 62 and 64, pages 101–3.

PRASARITA PADOTTANASANA I (SPREAD LEGS INTENSE FORWARD BEND) Use blocks if you need to; release head down completely. See Figures 72 and 73, pages 108–10.

HINDI SQUAT Either modified with props or the full pose. See Figures 62 and 64, pages 101–3.

SAVASANA (CORPSE POSE) Relax completely in classic or supported pose. See Figures 133–35, pages 155–57.

Completing Your Day

Evening or Before-Bed Practice

A routine conducive to relaxation works well in the late evening. At the end of the day, your body tends to be more supple simply because you have been moving around for several hours. Therefore this sequence will include plenty of forward bends.

SUKHASANA (EASY SEATED POSE) WITH TWIST On both sides of body. See Figures 80 and 81, pages 118–20.

JANUSIRSASANA (HEAD-TO-KNEE POSE) On both right and left sides. See Figures 84 and 85, pages 122–23.

CHATUSHPADA PITHAM (FOUR-LEGGED PLATFORM POSE) See Figures 86 and 87, pages 123–25.

APANASANA (KNEE-TO-CHEST POSE) Do complete series on each side. See Figures 23–26, pages 73–75.

DVIPADA PITHAM (TWO-LEGGED PLATFORM POSE) See Figures 19–22, pages 71–72.

APANASANA (BOTH KNEES-TO-CHEST POSE) Both knees at once. See Figures 29–31, pages 77–78.

NOTE: Either stop here or continue with the following sequence:

DANDASANA (STAFF POSE) See Figures 82 and 83, pages 120–21.

PASCHIMOTTANASANA (SEATED FORWARD BEND) See Figures 89 and 90, pages 125–27.

PURVOTTANASANA (FULL ANTERIOR STRETCH) See Figures 91 and 92, pages 127–29.

MARICHYASANA (SEATED TWISTED POSE) Do Stage 1 and/or Stage 2. See Figures 94 and 95, pages 130–31.

SUKHASANA (EASY SEATED POSE) with the Ujjayi breath (breath exercise #4, pages 52 and 53). See Figure 80, pages 118–20.

SAVASANA (CORPSE POSE) Relax completely. See Figures 133–35, pages 155–57.

PART 3

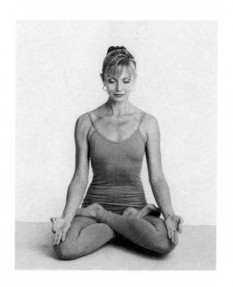

Completion

16

Let's Meditate

You now have both an intellectual understanding of yoga and a physical experience of this discipline. Having become familiar with the philosophical concepts and technical principles involved, you can breathe, position your body, and relax in ways that prepare you for the final phase of this journey called yoga.

Although you don't need to formally meditate in order to practice hatha yoga—nor is the practice of hatha yoga mandatory in order to meditate—the two practices support one another. Through your practice of yoga, you've enhanced both your abilities to concentrate and to relax—the two most important requirements for a meditation practice. This chapter will deepen your understanding of what meditation is, teach you its many benefits, and guide you in beginning a practice of your own.

What Is Meditation?

An exquisite methodology exists within the yoga tradition that is designed to reveal the interconnectedness of every living thing. This fundamental unity is referred to as *advaita.* Meditation is the actual experience of this union.

In *The Yoga Sutras,* Patañjali gives instructions on how to meditate and describes what factors constitute a meditation practice. The second sutra in the first chapter states that yoga (or union) happens when the mind becomes quiet. This mental stillness is created by bringing the body, mind, and senses into balance which, in turn, relaxes the nervous system. Patañjali goes on to explain that meditation begins when we discover that our never-ending quest to possess things and our continual craving for pleasure and security can never be satisfied. When we finally realize this, our external quest turns inward, and we have shifted into the realm of meditation.

By dictionary definition, "meditation" means to reflect upon, ponder, or contemplate. It can also denote a devotional exercise of contemplation or a contemplative discourse of a religious or philosophical nature. The word *meditate* comes from the Latin *meditari,* which means to think about or consider. *Med* is the root of this word and means "to take appropriate measures." In our culture, to meditate can be interpreted several ways. For instance, you might meditate on—or consider—a course of action regarding your child's education, or a career change that would entail a move across the country. Viewing a powerful movie or play, you may be moved to meditate upon—or ponder—the moral issues plaguing today's society.

In the yogic context, meditation, or *dhyana,* is defined more specifically as a state of pure consciousness. It is the seventh stage, or limb, of the yogic path and follows *dharana,* the art of concentration. Dhyana in turn precedes *samadhi,* the state of final liberation or enlightenment—the last step in Patañjali's eight-limbed system. These three limbs—dharana (concentration), dhyana (meditation), and samadhi (ecstasy)—are inextricably linked and collectively referred to as *samyama,* the inner practice, or subtle discipline, of the yogic path.

Recall that the first four limbs—yama (ethics), niyama (self-discipline), asana (posture), and pranayama (life-force extension)—are considered external disciplines. The fifth step, *pratyahara,* represents the withdrawal of the senses. This sensual withdrawal arises out of the practice of the first four steps and links the external to the internal. When we are grounded physically and mentally, we are keenly aware of our senses, yet disengaged at the same time. Without this ability to remain detached, yet observant, it is not possible to meditate. Even though you need to be able to concentrate in order to meditate, meditation is more than concentration. It ultimately evolves into an expanded state of awareness.

When we concentrate, we direct our mind toward what appears to be an object apart from ourselves. We become acquainted with this object and establish contact with it. To shift into the meditation realm, however, we need to become involved with this object; we need to communicate with it. The result of this exchange, of course, is a deep awareness that there is no difference between us (as the subject) and that which we concentrate or meditate upon (the object). This brings us to the state of samadhi, or self-realization.

A good way to understand this is to think about the development of a relationship. First, we meet someone—that is, we make contact. Then by spending time together, listening to, and sharing with one another, we develop a relationship. In the next stage, we merge with this person in the form of a deep friendship, partnership, or marriage. The "you" and "me" become an "us."

According to *The Yoga Sutras,* our pain and suffering is created by the misperception that we are separate from nature. The realization that we aren't separate may be experienced spontaneously, without effort. However, most of us need guidance. Patañjali's eight-limbed system provides us with the framework we need.

Ways to Meditate

Just as there are numerous styles of hatha yoga, so there are many ways to meditate. The first stage of meditation is to concentrate on a specific object or establish a point of focus, with the eyes either opened or closed. Silently repeating a word or phrase, audibly reciting a prayer or chant, visualizing an image such as a deity or, focusing on an object such as a lighted candle in front of you are all commonly recommended points of focus. Observing or counting your breaths and noticing bodily sensations are also optional focal points. Let's take a closer look.

The Use of Sound. *Mantra* yoga employs the use of a particular sound, phrase, or affirmation as a point of focus. The word *mantra* comes from *man,* which means "to think," and *tra,* which suggests "instrumentality." Therefore, *mantra* is an instrument of thought. It also has come to mean "protecting the person who receives it." Traditionally, you can only receive a mantra from a teacher, one who knows you and your particular needs. The act of repeating your mantra is called *japa,* which means recitation. Just as contemplative prayer and affirmation need to be stated with purpose and feeling, a mantra meditation practice requires conscious engagement on the part of the meditator. Maharishi Mahesh Yogi's Transcendental Meditation (TM) espouses the practice of mantra yoga.

Chanting, an extension of mantra yoga, is a powerful way to enter into meditation. Longer than a mantra, a chant involves both rhythm and pitch. Western traditions use chants and hymns to invoke the name of God, to inspire, and to produce a spiritual awakening. Dating back to Vedic times, Indian chanting comes out of a tradition that believes in the creative power of sound and its potential to transport us to an expanded state of awareness. The *rishis,* or ancient seers, taught that all of creation is a manifestation of the primordial sound *Om.* Reflected in an interpretation of the word *universe*—"one song"—*Om* is the seed sound of all other sounds. Chanting Sanskrit often and properly produces profound spiritual and physical effects.

Many beginners find using a mantra in their meditation very effective and relatively easy. Chanting, on the other hand, can be intimidating for some people. If you feel awkward chanting on your own, use one of the many audiotapes of chants on the market, or participate in a group meditation where a meditation teacher leads the chant and the students repeat it. Although chanting in Sanskrit can be very powerful, reciting a meaningful prayer or affirmation in any language can be effective.

The Use of Imagery. Visualizing is also a good way to meditate; one that beginners often find easy to practice. Traditionally, a meditator visualizes his or her chosen deity—a god or goddess—in vivid and detailed fashion. Essentially any object is valid.

Some practitioners visualize a natural object such as a flower or the ocean; others meditate on the chakras, or energy centers, in the body. In this type of meditation, you focus on the area or organ of the body corresponding to a particular chakra, imagining the particular color associated with it.

Gazing. Another variation on the use of imagery is to maintain an open-eyed focus upon an object. This focus is referred to as *drishti,* which means "view," "opinion," or "gaze." Again the choices available to you here are virtually limitless. Candle gazing is a popular form of this method. Focusing on a flower in a vase, or a statue, or picture of a deity are other possibilities.

Use this technique with your eyes fully opened or partially closed, creating a softer, diffused gaze. Many of the classical hatha yoga postures have gazing points, and the use of drishti is especially emphasized in the Ashtanga style of hatha yoga. Many pranayama techniques also call for specific positioning of the eyes, such as gazing at the "third eye"—the point between the eyebrows—or at the tip of the nose.

Breathing. Using the breath as a point of focus is yet another possibility. You can do this by actually counting the breaths like you would in pranayama practice.

Ultimately, however, meditating on the breath just means purely observing the breath as it is, without changing it in any way. In this instance, the breath becomes the sole object of your meditation. You observe every nuance of the breath and each sensation it produces: how it moves in your abdomen and torso, how it feels as it moves in and out of your nose, its quality, its temperature, and so on. Though you are fully aware of all these details, you don't dwell on them or judge them in any way; you remain detached from what you're observing. What you discover is neither good nor bad; you simply allow yourself to be with the breath from moment to moment.

Breath observance is the predominant technique used by practitioners of *vipassana,* commonly referred to as "insight" or "mindfulness" meditation. Popularized by such renowned teachers as Thich Nhat Hanh, Jack Kornfield, and Jon Kabat-Zinn, this is a form of Buddhist practice. The word *vipassana,* which literally means "to see clearly" or "look deeply," is also interpreted to mean "the place where the heart dwells," and reflects the premise that thought arises out of our hearts.

Physical Sensations. Another way to meditate is to watch a physical sensation. Practice this with the same degree of detail as you would when watching the breath. In this context, you will look deeply at, or penetrate, a particular sensation that draws your attention, such as how hot or cool your hands feel. The increased sensitivity you gained due to your asana practice may provide you with other points of focus: the strength of your spine or the suppleness you feel in your lower body, for example. Observing a particular emotion or any specific area of discomfort is also a possibility. Whatever you choose remains your point of focus for the whole practice. You may find that observing a physical sensation—becoming keenly aware of all its intricacies and yet remaining detached—can be more challenging than observing the breath. For most beginners, mantras, chants, and visualizations offer more tangible ways to replace or calm the scattered thoughts of our minds, which seem to be perpetually on sensory overload.

Meditation Postures

Sitting. Although you can meditate—or become fully absorbed—in any activity or position of stillness, sitting is the most commonly recommended posture. There are a number of classic seated poses, but Sukhasana (Easy Seated Pose) is

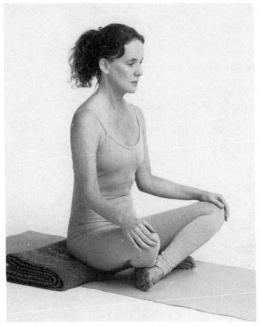

FIG. 136

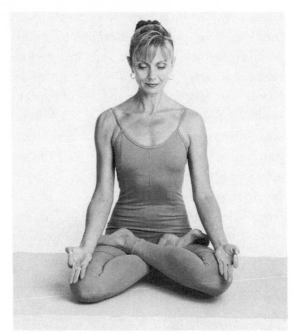

FIG. 137

obviously the most basic. (Figure 136.) More flexible meditators prefer Padmasana (Lotus Pose). (Figure 137.)

Sitting in a chair also works. (Figure 138.) It's no less effective and certainly no less spiritual, and it's often the best choice for beginners. The most important things are that your spine remain upright and that you feel steady and comfortable—the same two qualities necessary for performing asanas. To maximize comfort on the floor, place a cushion or folded blanket under your buttocks to elevate them and gently guide your knees down toward the floor. This helps support the natural lumbar curve of the lower back. Some people prefer kneeling "Japanese-style." (Figure 139.) There are also small, slanted wooden benches for this position.

Relax your arms and place your hands on your thighs or in your lap, with the palms in a relaxed position either facing up or down. Roll your shoulders back and down and gently lift the chest. Keep your neck long and the chin tilted slightly downward. Depending upon which technique you are following, the eyes may be opened or closed. Breathing is natural and free.

Walking. A moving meditation—highly recommended by many teachers—may be an enjoyable option for you. The challenge of this form is to walk slowly and consciously, each step becoming your focal point. Destination, distance, and pace are all incidental. Relax your arms at your sides and move freely, coordinating your breath with your steps. For instance, you might breathe in for 3 steps and breathe out for 3 steps. If that feels awkward or difficult, just breathe freely. Although you can practice walking meditation anywhere, choose a setting you particularly love—the ocean, a favorite park, or a meadow. Remember, getting somewhere is not the issue. Rather, the complete involvement in the act of walking becomes your meditation.

Standing. Standing is another meditation practice that can be very powerful. It is often recommended for those practitioners who find sitting difficult, and martial artists find that it builds physical, mental, and spiritual strength. Stand with your feet hip- to shoulder-distance apart. Knees are soft; arms rest comfortably at your sides. Check to see that the whole body is aligned in good posture: shoulders rolled back and down, chest open, neck long, head floating on top, and chin parallel to the floor. Either keep your eyes opened or softly close them.

Reclining. Even though lying down is associated with relaxation, the classic corpse posture, Savasana, is also used for meditation. Lie down on your back with your arms at your sides, palms facing upward. (Figure 140.) Touch

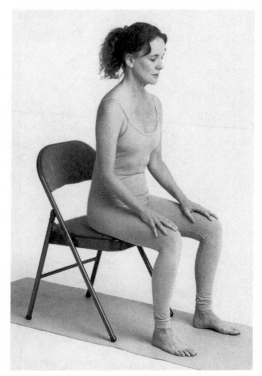

FIG. 138

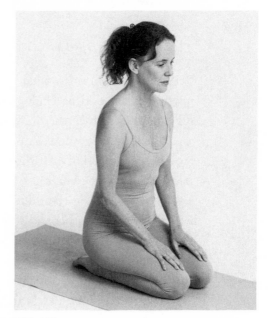

FIG. 139

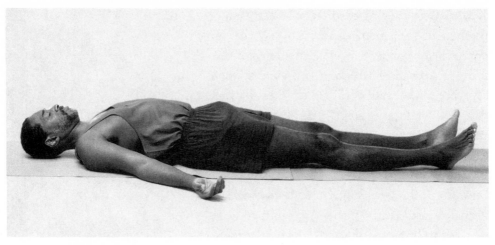

FIG. 140

your heels together and allow the feet to fall away from one another, completely relaxed. Although your eyes may be opened or closed, some people find it easier to stay awake with their eyes open. A supine meditation, although more physically restful than other positions, entails a greater degree of alertness to remain awake and focused. Therefore, beginners may find it more difficult to meditate in this position without falling asleep.

The Benefits of Meditation

Research has confirmed what the yogis of ancient times already knew: Profound physiological—and psychological—changes take place when we meditate, causing an actual shift in the brain and in the involuntary processes of the body.

This is how it works. An instrument called an electroencephalograph (EEG) records mental activity. During waking activity, when the mind constantly moves from one thought to another, the EEG registers jerky and rapid lines categorized as *beta* waves. When the mind calms down through meditation, the EEG shows waves that are smoother and slower, and categorizes them as *alpha* waves. As meditation deepens, brain activity decreases even further. The EEG then registers an even smoother, slower pattern of activity we call *theta* waves. Studies on meditators have shown decreased perspiration and a slower rate of respiration accompanied by a decrease of metabolic wastes in the bloodstream. Lower blood pressure and an enhanced immune system are further benefits noted by research studies.

The health benefits meditation produces naturally reflect the mental and physical effects of this process. At the very least, meditation teaches you how to manage stress; reducing stress in turn enhances your overall physical health and emotional well-being. On a deeper level, it can add to the quality of your life by teaching you to be fully alert, aware, and alive. In short, it is a celebration of your self. You are not meditating to get anything, but rather to look at and let go of anything you do not need.

17

Starting Your Own
Meditation Practice

We highly recommend a period of daily meditation. Add it to the end of your asana practice, or set aside another block of time. The important thing is that you find a time that works best for you. Don't do too much too soon; you're apt to get discouraged and stop all together.

When and Where to Practice

To establish consistency, meditate at the same time and in the same place every day. Choose a place that is quiet, one that is pleasant, where you'll be undisturbed.

Traditionally, the morning is considered the optimal time because you are less likely to be distracted by the demands of your day. Many people find that a morning meditation helps them enter the day with a greater degree of equanimity and poise. However, if a morning practice is a struggle, try an afternoon or early evening meditation.

If you are new to yoga and meditation, you may find adding 5 or 10 minutes of meditation at the end of your asana practice is enough. When meditating independently of your yoga practice, a 15- to 20-minute time frame seems manageable for most beginners.

Posture

Choose a position that works for you. If you prefer sitting, either on a chair or on the floor, keep the spine erect and the body relaxed. Your hands should rest comfortably on your lap or thighs, with the palms up or down. If you choose to walk or stand, maintaining good posture is also critical, with your arms hanging freely by your sides. When lying down, place yourself in a symmetrical and comfortable position with the appropriate support under your head and knees if needed.

Method

Decide on your point of focus. If sound appeals to you, create your own mantra, silently or audibly repeating a word or phrase that is calming to you, such as "peace," "love," or "joy."

Affirmations also work. "I am relaxed" or "I am calm and alert" are excellent. Think "I am" as you breathe in and "relaxed" or "calm and alert" as you breathe out. Using a tape of chants or listening to a relaxing piece of music are also options. (See Resources.)

If you choose imagery, visualize your favorite spot in nature with your eyes closed, or gaze upon an object placed in front of you: a lighted candle, a flower, or a picture of your favorite saint or deity.

One way to observe the breath is to count it: Breathe in for 3 to 7 counts and breathe out for the same length of time. Then shift to simply observing the breath, noticing its own natural rhythm and its movement in your torso.

Whichever posture and method you choose, stick with them for the duration of your meditation period. Indeed, once you find what works for you, you'll want to maintain that practice indefinitely.

Do not be surprised or discouraged by how frequently your thoughts wander. When you realize that your mind has become distracted, simply return to your chosen point of focus.

How Do You Know If It's Working?

At the beginning you might feel uncomfortable meditating—sitting for 20 minutes may cause your legs to fall asleep or cramp up, walking slowly may bring up feelings of impatience or agitation, and reclining poses may merely make you fall asleep. Conversely, you may have some profound experiences the first few times you sit, only to spend the next few frustrating days trying to duplicate them. Relax. Meditation shouldn't cause you to feel unreasonably stressed or physically uncomfortable. If it does, reduce the length of your practice time or change your position (from walking to sitting; from sitting to standing). If that doesn't work, go back to incorporating a few minutes of meditation into your asana practice instead of holding onto a formal practice. After a few days, try returning to your normal meditation routine.

If you continue having trouble with your meditation practice, you may need to seek the guidance of an experienced teacher or the support of a group that meets regularly to meditate together. Indications of your progress, with or without a teacher or group, are feelings of mental calm and physical comfort, and the ability to be present in all your experiences.

Power of Love Meditation

The power of love is universally recognized and has been used by the ancient healing traditions in cultures throughout the world. Today, Western physicians acknowledge its benefits to the immune system, while psychologists agree that it does wonders for mental health. Both the yoga and Buddhist teachings provide us with meditations designed to free ourselves of negative emotions which interfere with our ability to love.

This battle of the heart is dramatically represented in the *Bhagavad Gita,* a classic Indian story about the conflict between two families. Although that conflict appears to be a conflict against external enemies, it is really the internal battle we wage within our own hearts.

Patañjali's thirty-third sutra describes a four-part process of clearing the heart of impure thoughts as a way to quiet the mind. He advises cultivating *maitri* (friendliness) toward pleasure and friends; *karuna* (compassion) for those who are in pain or suffering, yourself included; *mudita* (rejoicing) or joyful acknowledgment of the noble or holy ones (including those who have helped you, those you admire, and your family); and *upeksanam* (indifference) to unholiness—in other words, equanimity toward those who have harmed you. As you can see, collectively these four stages sound remarkably like the "Love thy neighbor as thyself" sentiment we're all familiar with.

The following instructions guide you through a full meditation which includes the fourfold stages or attitudes Patañjali taught in his *Yoga Sutras.* It is both practical and profound. With regular practice, this meditation will guide you toward a better relationship with yourself, those you are close to, and the world around you.

Loving Your Enemies Meditation

This meditation will take anywhere from 5 to 20 minutes, or even longer if you wish. The important thing is to be comfortable with it. You don't really need to time yourself. However, we recommend staying in Stages 1 and 2 for 1 to 2 minutes each; in Stage 3 for 3 to 5 minutes; and in Stage 4 for 5 to 15 minutes.

1. Get into a comfortable, seated position, either in a chair with your legs uncrossed, or on the floor. Adjust your posture so that your spine is upright, yet your body feels relaxed. Rest your hands in your lap or on your thighs, with the palms either facing up or down.

2. Close your eyes and bring your attention to your breathing. Take a few conscious and deep abdominal breaths. Let your exhalations carry out any tension or anxiety you're feeling now, and use them throughout your meditation to expel any tension or anxiety that comes up.

   If it is helpful, you may use the previously recommended affirmations—"I am" on the in-breath and "calm and relaxed" on the out-breath—to center yourself during this practice.

3. Bring your awareness to your heart. Allow your breaths to massage this area. Notice any specific feelings or thoughts you may have about yourself, people you know, or any particular event. Cultivate a detached and nonjudgmental attitude to anything that comes up for you.

4. Continue to focus on the heart area while doing the following:

   • Cultivate a friendly and accepting attitude toward yourself and your friends;
   • Develop feelings of compassion and understanding for all those who suffer;
   • Be joyful in your thoughts about a particular person who's important to you or a saint or guru you hold in high esteem;

- Maintain feelings of indifference and equanimity to anyone who has harmed you or anyone else. Don't get sucked into their mean-spiritedness or harmful deeds.

5. To complete your meditation, take 3 to 5 deep abdominal breaths. Open your eyes and slowly get up.

Allow the focus of this meditation to be the fourfold stages of opening your heart in order to clear your mind. Realize, however, that it also incorporates other elements common to all forms of meditation: choosing a stable and comfortable position, awareness of breath, use of affirmation, and imagery. It's all right if only one of the stages dominates the meditation. For example, you may be drawn to the concern for a friend who is in pain, or you may want to focus on the life's work of someone who inspires you. No better advice can be given here than to—literally—listen to your heart!

Namasté

Namasté, the traditional expression of greeting and farewell practiced among yogis, is performed with the hands placed in prayer position at the heart center. It is usually accompanied with a bowing of the head and body. It means "The Divine in me salutes the Divine in you."

Resources

Yoga Journal
2054 University Avenue
Berkeley, CA 94704
(510) 841-9200
(510) 644-3101 fax
For subscriptions: (800) I-DO-YOGA
For books and tapes: (800) I-DO-YOGA
(436-9642)

YOGA STYLES

Iyengar/B. K. S. Iyengar
B. K. S. Iyengar Yoga National
Association of the United States, Inc.
(800) 889-YOGA (9642)

Ashtanga Yoga/K. Pattabhi Jois
Beryl Bender Birch and Tom Birch
(Power Yoga)
The Hard and the Soft
325 E. 41st Street, #203
New York, NY 10017-5916
(212) 661-2895

Richard Freeman
3020 Jefferson Street
Boulder, CO 80304
(303) 449-6102

Tim Miller
Ashtanga Yoga Center
118 West E Street
Encinitas, CA 92024
(760) 632-7093

Viniyoga/T. K. V. Desikachar
Martin and Margaret Pierce
The Pierce Program
1164 N. Highland Ave., NE
Atlanta, GA 30306
(404) 875-7110

Gary Kraftsow
1030 E. Kuiaha Road
Haiku, HI 96708
(808) 572-1414
(808) 572-5775 fax

Richard Miller, Ph.D.
Anahata Press
1111 Grandview Road
Sebastapol, CA 95472
(415) 456-3909

Kundalini Yoga/Yogi Bhajan
International Kundalini Yoga Teachers
Association
Route 2, Box 4, Shady Lane
Espanola, NM 87532
(505) 753-0423
(505) 753-5982 fax

Kripalu Yoga/Yogi Amrit Desai
Kripalu Center for Yoga and Health
P.O. Box 793, West Street
Lenox, MA 01240-0793
(800) 741-7353
(413) 448-3152
(413) 448-3384 fax

Ananda Yoga/Swami Kriyananda
The Expanding Light
14618 Tyler Foote Road
Nevada City, CA 95959
(800) 346-5350
(916) 478-7518
(916) 478-7519 fax

Yoga College of India—Choudhury
Yoga/Bikram Choudhury
Yoga College of India
8800 Wilshire Boulevard, 2nd Fl.
Beverly Hills, CA 90211
(310) 854-5800
(310) 854-6200 fax

Integral Yoga/Swami Satchidananda
Satchidananda Ashram–Yogaville
Route 1, Box 1720
Buckingham, VA 23921
(800) 858-YOGA (9642)
(804) 969-3121
(804) 969-1303 fax

Sivananda Yoga/Swami Vishnu-devananda
Sivananda Yoga Vedanta Center
243 W. 24th Street
New York, NY 10011
(800) 783-YOGA (9642)
(212) 255-4560
(212) 727-7392 fax

Index